COMMONSENSE PAEDIATRICS

Presented to

----

with the compliments of

----

your Upjohn Representative

As a service to medical education Upjohn

'It will be gathered from this that the physician who undertakes the investigation of the early stages of disease must not only be a man of wide experience but must have trained himself to observe on lines that have hitherto received little attention. The training, amongst other things, must have included the watching of patients for long periods to see the outcome of the complaint. If this is grasped, it will be understood how vain it is to expect the early stages to be revealed in hospitals, where the custom is to hand the out-patient department over to the junior physician who lacks that experience which should make him a competent examiner. I have for many years been calling attention to this error in education and showing how it hampers practice and research.'

Sir James MacKenzie, 1920

'We need the whole physician for the whole patient' *Plato*

COMMONSENSE PAEDIATRICS

Dr Margaret Pollak

Reader in Developmental Paediatrics
Hon. Consultant Paediatrician
Director, Sheldon Children's Centre
King's College Hospital, London

and

Dr John Fry

General Practitioner,
Beckenham, Kent

with a chapter by
Dr Peter Robson
Senior Lecturer in Paediatric Neurology
King's College Hospital, London

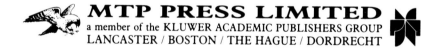

MTP PRESS LIMITED
a member of the KLUWER ACADEMIC PUBLISHERS GROUP
LANCASTER / BOSTON / THE HAGUE / DORDRECHT

Published in the UK and Europe by
MTP Press Limited
Falcon House
Lancaster, England

British Library Cataloguing in Publication Data

Pollak, Margaret
  Commonsense paediatrics.
  1. Pediatrics
  I. Title   II. Fry, John, *1922–*
  618.92   RJ45

ISBN 0-85200-945-3

Published in the USA by
MTP Press
A division of Kluwer Boston Inc
190 Old Derby Street
Hingham, MA 02043, USA

Library of Congress Cataloging in Publication Data

Pollak, Margaret.
  Commonsense paediatrics.

  Includes bibliographies and index.
  1. Pediatrics.   I. Fry, John.   II. Title.
III. Title: Common sense paediatrics. [DNLM:
Pediatrics. WS 100 P771c]
RJ45.P55 1986   618.92   86-2929
ISBN 0-85200-945-3

Typeset and printed by
Butler & Tanner Ltd, Frome and London

Contents

Section IV SOCIETY, FAMILY AND COMMUNITY

Section V USES OF . . .

Section VI THE WHOLE CHILD

Preface

As 'seasoned campaigners' we offer our readers more than 60 joint practice years of commonsense experience on children and their problems.

Child care is a large and fascinating part of general family practice. More than any other discipline it is a mix of understanding the wide range of normal and abnormal development, of skilful diagnosis and treatment of treatable conditions, of long-term care for handicapped children, and of organizing and carrying out prevention.

For all this and more the physician has to rely on sound knowledge and understanding of the child, parents, family, social and community conditions, available services and the likely natural history of the condition – and to dispense all this with humanity, sense and sensibility.

We have divided the book logically into 6 sections:

(1) Factual background.
(2) Universal problems of behaviour and development.
(3) Common clinical disorders, so frequent and yet often so difficult to manage.
(4) Social, family and community factors that create and influence many problems of childhood.
(5) How to use available services and resources with discrimination and sensitivity.
(6) The importance of understanding and managing the whole child.

We have no single group of readers in mind. We hope that our views will be appreciated, for example, by parents, nurses, health visitors, general practitioners, community physicians and paediatricians – in fact all who care for children.

MARGARET POLLAK
JOHN FRY

SECTION I

First Principles

1

Children in the practice

BASIC FACTS

In an average practice in a typical area care for children takes up about one third of a general practitioner's work.

They live within families in their homes with various social, genetic and cultural factors influencing their health, disease patterns and even risks of dying, albeit rarely now. As a backcloth it is important to appreciate how many children there are, from what problems and diseases they suffer and the work they create for medical services.

How many?

One quarter of the *population* is under 15 years of age (Figure 1.1). Therefore, in a general practice of 2000 persons there will be 500 children. These 500 will be equally distributed.

166 will be 0–4 years old
167 will be 5–9 years old
167 will be 10–15 years old

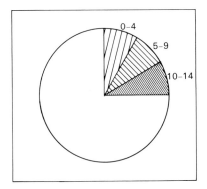

Figure 1.1   Age distribution in a general practice.

Each year 26 children will be *born* in the practice. Of these up to ten will be to primipara. 10% of babies are now delivered by Caesarean section and about 20% by forceps.

The *infant mortality rate* (10 per 1000 in 1983) is such that there may be one infant death every 4 years. The rates are higher in inner cities, in lower social groups and in other at-risk groups.

Of babies born now, boys can *expect to live* for 75 years and girls for 80 years.

What problems?

'Problems' can be divided into mortality, general morbidity, chronic diseases and handicaps.

In a practice (J.F.) with 500 children, the following rates and numbers can be expected.

Mortality

After the first year of life, there should be only one death in children (1–15 years) approximately once every 10 years or so.

The chief causes of deaths in children (0–15 years), are, in order (Figure 1.2):

birth trauma	(33%)
congenital defects	(20%)
infections	(17%)
accidents	(15%)
neoplasms	(5%)
others	(10%)

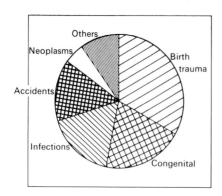

Figure 1.2　Chief causes of mortality in children.

Morbidity

Generally, children now are, or should be, healthy. The conditions for which they are brought to the general practitioner tend to be minor.

The content of morbidity varies with the age of the child:

at 0–1 years
    1–4 years
    5–9 years
   10–14 years

(Figure 1.3 shows percentage proportions of consultations at these ages for various reasons.)

Chronic conditions

These are important because they require careful assessment and long-term care.

In a general population of 2000, the following are numbers that may be expected of the 500 children who have or have had chronic or recurring disorders.

Recurring disorders	Number
Asthma	25
(but 125 children will have had one or more attacks of 'acute wheezy chests')	
Eczema	50
Epilepsy	4
Enuresis	100 at 5 years
	30 at 10 years
	5 at 15 years
Squint	15
Recurring headaches	60
Recurring abdominal pains	30
Behaviour problems	25
Severe physical handicap	2
Minor–moderate handicap	20
(Note the high rates of possible psychosomatic disorders)	

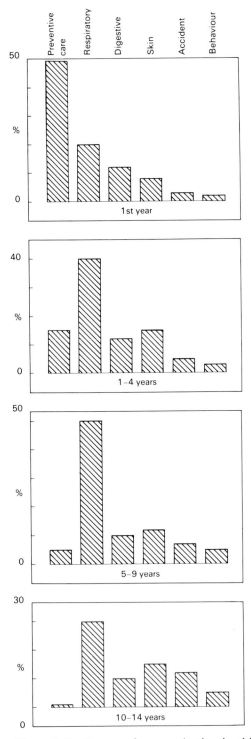

Figure 1.3 Reasons for consultation in children of various ages.

Chronic conditions (at 7–11 years)	%
Recurrent headaches – abdominal pains	36
Eczema	20
Enuresis	12
Behaviour	10
Asthma	8
Physical handicap	8
Squint	5
Epilepsy	1
	100

Consultation rates

General practice

In a practice (JF)

Over 90% of children under 5 years consult their GP annually for all services including prevention.

64% of children 5–15 years consult their GP annually.

The annual consultation rates per child are highest in the first year and then decline, but are up in the first school years (Figure 1.4). (The annual consultation rate for the whole practice is 3.5.)

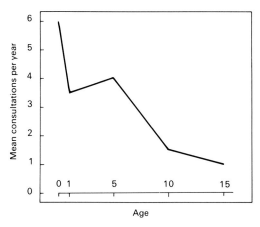

Figure 1.4 Average annual consultation rates per child.

Health Visitors

Court[1] reported that the annual number of health visitor visits/contacts per child were:

under 1 year	12
1–2 years	4
2–4 years	2
Total	18 per child under 5

Morbidity

Morbidity as shown by proportions of consultations for disease groups (Figure 1.5) is:

respiratory disorders	40%
infections	12%
skin	10%
accidents	7%
gastrointestinal	6%
behavioural	3%
genitourinary	2%
'symptoms'	3%
(prophylactic)	10%
others	7%
	100%

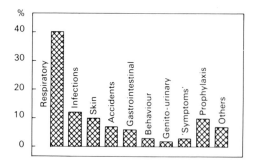

Figure 1.5   Reasons for consultation in children.

Hospital

In general children are referred to hospital less than adults but it is possible that 1 in 5 will attend a hospital service in any year.

Percentages of children and adults attending a hospital service in 1 year

	Children[1] (%)	Adults[2] (%)
Admitted to hospital	7	12
Referred to outpatient departments	2	18
Attend accident emergency departments	15	20

Admissions

One half of childrens' admissions are for 'emergencies'. The disease groups causing admission were[1]:

respiratory	21%
trauma	17%
congenital and perinatal	15%
symptoms	10%
gastrointestinal	9%
eyes and ears	8%
other infections	5%
genitourinary	4%
others	11%

The numbers of surgical admissions for an average size general practice in 1 year would be:

tonsillectomy, adenoidectomy and ear surgery	15
hernia, testes, hydrocoeles	10
squint	1
others	5

Outpatients and accident–emergency departments

Percentages of those attending were[1]:

accidents	22
'symptoms'	12
congenital and perinatal	10
respiratory	8
infections	7
tonsils/adenoids	6
ear	6
eye	6
skin	6
gastrointestinal	6
genitourinary	4
mental	2
others	5
	100

Social problems

Morbidity is incomplete, without the social component being appreciated. In the practice of 2000 persons there is much social pathology that can have serious effects on children.

The social problems per 2000 are[3]:

poverty (families on supplementary benefits with children)	100+
unemployed	250+
one parent families	40
juvenile delinquents	10
children in care	4

BASIC PRINCIPLES

Is the child really ill?

Children cannot communicate easily with doctors and nurses. The first decision a parent, doctor or nurse has to make is whether the child is ill and if so, how ill.

Most, but not all, children who are really ill are:

floppy
quiet
still
listless
give the doctor a feeling of anxiety and unease even with the first
   look – and the 'first look assessment' takes an increasing importance with experience.

Jane R. age 2
The adored only child of publicans.
   A frequent attender for less than real medical reasons. Mother–
child relationship poor.
   Jane usually screamed, kicked and resisted attempts at exami-
nation.
   Late Saturday evening a home visit was requested as Jane had
been 'off colour' for 2 days.
   On arrival mother was busy in a full bar. In a back room Jane
was lying still and quiet. No screams or resistance on examination
of a tender and distended abdomen. She looked sick.
   Admitted to hospital and a perforated appendix was removed.

Hyperactive 'surgery wreckers' are rarely seriously physically ill. It
may be part of their 'normal' behaviour or a sign of poor mother–
child control and relationship.
   Screaming children are rarely seriously ill. Their behaviour tends to
mirror their home environment and their parents' lack of control of
a wilful independent personality passing through the negative period
between 1 and 3 years.
   Try to differentiate between crying which is purposeful and
reasonable and screaming which is temper and unreasonable. Examination is sometimes impossible but fortunately there are few abnormalities in the screamers.
   Crying children may be sick or unhappy. The parents, too, may be
unhappy for obvious or hidden reasons.
   The sick child may cry from pain or discomfort arising from causes
to be remembered as:

earache
in apparent trauma, accidental or non-accidental

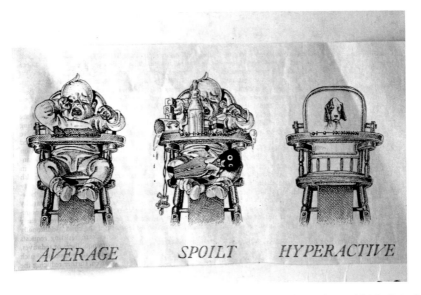

Figure 1.6 The hyperactive child (by kind permission of *World Medicine*).

abdominal pains from non-serious colic, constipation or gastroenteritis
urinary tract infections
strangulated hernia
torsion of testis
intussusception
osteomyelitis

What is wrong?

In an *ideal situation* a leisurely history is obtained and an examination carried out in a relaxed atmosphere. A definitive diagnosis is made and specific treatment applied successfully. Parents are impressed and satisfied.

In *real life*, the sick child is unwell and unhappy, feverish and 'off food'. No physical abnormalities are detected. No definite diagnosis is possible. No specific curative treatment is indicated. The condition takes a few days to recover naturally. Parents are unimpressed.

Beware of making a *'pseudo diagnosis'* and prescribing pseudo treatment. It is far better to be honest with the parents and with oneself, not to attempt to make a diagnosis and yet retain their co-operation, confidence and respect.

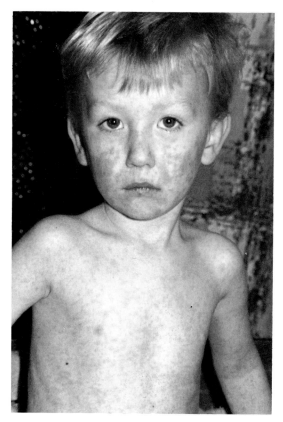

Figure 1.7 Measles.

Parents with a sick child are naturally distressed, worried and fearful of the worst. A clear, calm explanation and reassurance, advice on how to relieve symptoms and arrangements to reassess the situation in a day or two, with availability sooner if necessary – such management cements a good doctor–patient relationship.

Probably the most important part of such care is *continuity of responsibility* with explanation of likely course and outcome, with promise to see the child again and with an emergency phone number.

Above all treat *parents as part of the caring team* and as sensible, co-operative and intent to do their best – unless there is evidence to the contrary.

The doctor should consider why the parents have come at this particular time? What are their fears? What are their expectations?

Nigel, 11 years
Brought by his capable mother because of headaches for the past week. Mother has always been considered as 'sensible'.

Seen by the junior partner who finds 'nil abnormal' on physical examination. To maintain his professional reputation he makes a diagnosis of *'sinusitis'*. X-rays of sinuses are ordered and are reported as normal.

Headaches continue. Junior partner now says that 'it must be *migraine'* and prescribes tablets.

It is now 3 weeks later and parents are concerned and disillusioned. They consult senior partner who knows Nigel and family well. Still there are no abnormal physical signs. Mother and Nigel cry during the consultation. Senior partner is disturbed by such unusual behaviour. No diagnosis is made but persisting headache for a month in a fit 11-year-old with no previous history has to be taken seriously.

Referral to specialist and investigations reveal a *frontal astrocytoma*.

Parents blame the young partner for making two wrong diagnoses and delaying referral.

It would have been better to make no diagnosis when none was apparent and to adopt open-minded 'wait and see' approach.

Fortunately, much more often the causes of 'I don't know' (IDK) diagnoses are benign such as:
minor self-limiting viral infections
exanthemata in prodromal stages
the 'presenting child syndrome' where the major problems lie in the mother and not the child.

Special difficulties

We all have our own special difficulties in caring for children in general. One of us, doing first locum in general practice, had not yet developed skills in examining children. Many children came with sore throats etc. On examination of throats, most children began screaming and arching necks, therefore, when the raw doctor tested for neck stiffness, all necks were stiff! Local hospital received more than usual number of admissions ?meningitis, until the new doctor learned a better technique for inspecting throats. It has, however, left her with a fear of missing early meningitis. We have vulnerable clinical 'blind spots' that can cause uncertainty and worry.

Difficulties are compounded by special factors:

second-hand history from mothers with variable degrees of observation and reporting.

few abnormal specific physical signs in many childrens' illnesses, particularly in early stages.

normal abnormalities in children. With the huge range of normality many apparent abnormalities may in fact be within normal limits.
catarrhal child syndrome
umbilical hernia
non-retractable foreskin
sticky eyes
tongue-tie
hydrocoele
orthopaedic conditions
(see Chapter 20)

Avoid radical treatments for self-limiting conditions such as large tonsils and adenoids.

Look for the '*cry wolf*' situation with an over-anxious mother who is a frequent attender for many minor problems. The child can, and may well, suffer from a serious disease.

Among examples of clinical pitfalls into which it is possible to fall are:

(1) *Congenital dislocation of hips* because of failure to repeat checks during infancy.

(2) *Meningitis in infants* because of paucity of classical signs. The child with meningitis may only be listless, dozy and feverish. Neck stiffness, tense fontanelle and rash may be absent.

Baby Y aged 3 months
Doctor (MP) called because baby was 'off feeds'.

Non-febrile, apparently well. MP suggested giving feed to observe.

During the feed transient facial and left arm spasm noted. Admitted to hospital where meningoccal meningitis diagnosed and treated with full recovery.

If feed had not been observed, diagnosis would have been delayed.

---

(3) A young child with *acute appendicitis* is not able to complain of shifting abdominal pain and localized tenderness in right iliac fossa. The child vomits, is generally unwell, may have diarrhoea and there may be vague general abdominal tenderness and distension. (See story of Jane on p. 11.)

(4) Beware of diagnosing fleeting pink rashes as *'German measles'*. Most are not true rubella. Apart from causing much anxiety in pregnant friends it is a slack diagnosis. Mothers sometimes state that their child had been diagnosed with 'German measles' two, three or four times. *Roseola* tricks everyone, with a feverish sick child for 3–4 days, worried parents and uncertain doctor, then rash and rapid recovery.

(5) Beware of over-diagnosing *Down's syndrome*, or other major congenital disorders by the infant's facial appearance. Look well at the parents – there may be family likenesses. Nevertheless, the initial diagnosis of Down's is often made from the face.

(6) Not all *enuresis* is functional and/or emotional. Always test urine to avoid missing major urological disorders.

(7) Beware of *loose pseudo diagnoses*. Seek evidence to confirm diagnosis of 'simple' problems.

   'growing pains' may delay diagnosis of juvenile rheumatoid disease.

   'teething', even if gums do look sore with erupting teeth, does not cause fever or general disturbances.

   'colic' or *'wind'* may be result of sucking for too long at empty breast or bottle, small teat or excessive gulping. Evening 3-month colic does occur and is resistant to therapy and advice but ceases spontaneously.

   'milk allergies' are very rare and have to be proven before diagnoses.

   'heart murmurs' – most soft systolic murmurs are benign and transient. A normal chest X-ray and absence of features of heart failure confirm.

(8) *Beware of missing* potentially dangerous conditions such as:

   epiglottitis as cause of croup
   fibrocystic disease as reason for non-thriving

16

deafness masking as mental retardation or behaviour problems
congenital dislocation of hips as reason for lateness in walking
undescended testes in a fat child
non-accidental injuries in a 'nice family'
mental retardation masking as a behaviour problem.

BASIC PRINCIPLES

Social class factors

The contributions of modern medical technologies in preventing disease and improving health have been less than the benefits of social advances and advantages that have become more evenly distributed throughout our society.

Old-time mass-killers such as smallpox, tuberculosis, rheumatic fever, scarlet fever, diphtheria, measles and gastroenteritis have been eliminated or much reduced in the UK (but still cause many deaths in developing countries) (Figure 1.8).

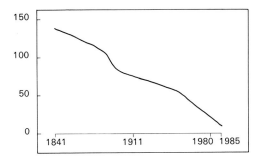

Figure 1.8 Reduction in mortality 1841–1985.

The health of children is closely related to their families, their environment and their culture. Good child care must always take note of these factors in prevention and management.

Classification of social class by the occupation of the breadwinner is a useful though crude delineation.

Mortality

Infant mortalities almost double from social classes 1 and 2 to social class 5 (Figure 1.9). Infant mortality is higher in illegitimate births

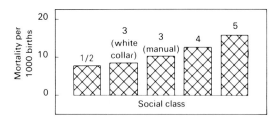

Figure 1.9 Infant mortality by social class (from reference 4).

(15.2) than legitimate (10.2). Fatal accidents in children are five times higher in social classes 4 and 5 than in social classes 1 and 2.

Chronic sickness

In children under 14 chronic sickness is also related to social class (Figure 1.10).

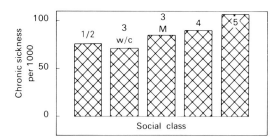

Figure 1.10 Chronic sickness in children by social class.

Use of health services (GP consultations)

There is an inverse relation between social class and use of GP services (Figure 1.11). The same trends apply to hospital and social services. Medical services as a whole are used more by socially disadvantaged

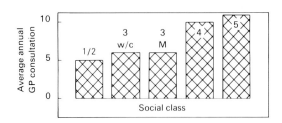

Figure 1.11 Average annual GP consultation by social class (from reference 5).

children. Preventive services are used more by higher social classes. Acute services are used more by lower social classes.

Non-use of immunization

Children of lower social groups are less likely to be immunized (Figure 1.12).

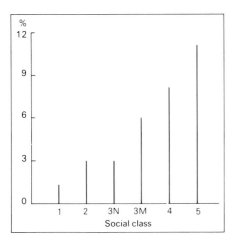

Figure 1.12 Non-use of diphtheria/polio immunization by social class (from reference 6).

Fulfilment of potential

More 16–19 year-olds of upper social classes fulfil their higher educational potential (Figure 1.13).

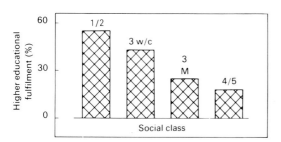

Figure 1.13 Higher education fulfilment by social class.

Family

The family influences that affect a child's health and behaviour are:

mother/child relationship: essential for psychological growth and well-being. The need for love, affection and self-esteem is a child's first requirement and stems from this relationship.

father/mother relationship: children are very sensitive to marital discord and to differences in parental views of child-rearing practices.

involvement of in-laws: dominant in-laws can seriously affect a mother's or a father's relationship with a child.

grannies (and child-minders): experienced and can be helpful but may force old fashioned views and remedies on to parents.

family feuds and views: younger children are highly susceptible to parents' views of other people and politics; children tend to take same attitudes to say, Northern Ireland, Jews and Arabs, gang warfare, political parties, etc. as their parents.

position of child in family: all positions have different significance. Eldest most independent, young often spoilt, middle one may be left out.

sibling relationships: often quite unknown to doctor and parents. Family relations test is useful for discovering unsuspected jealousies, admirations, etc.

sickness in the family: depressed parents have little time for children. A sick parent leads to extra family roles for the other parent. A sick father means less income and fewer amenities. Disability may mean inability to play with children or take them out.

working parents in poor housing cannot manage a child's general needs and illness as well as those in good housing and amenities.

some parents in social classes 4 and 5 are poor copers with life in general and with health services in particular.

with smaller families and fewer children, each child is precious and parental desires to maximize abilities and achieve perfection are greater. Demands and expectations of health services are likely to increase.

Imagine a working mother collects her child from the nursery on her way home from work. At home a meal needs cooking, other children and her husband make demands on her. The home may need heating. She notices the child is hot and fractious. She goes to the GP's surgery and waits her turn. She is given a prescription which then needs obtaining from the chemist. A sick child needs helping. It is 'all too much'. How much easier to go to the Casualty department where a junior doctor may even admit the child overnight.

Environment

Some examples of the effects of environment are:

town: much traffic, restricted safe playing space.

country: remote and isolated and has to travel to friends.

high rise dwellers: enforced isolation.

new town blues: loss of relatives and friends. New neighbours of similar age and same problems and difficulties.

isolated mums: depressed, little easy ready-made opportunities for social intercourse.

cultures: different child-rearing patterns and different family relationships.

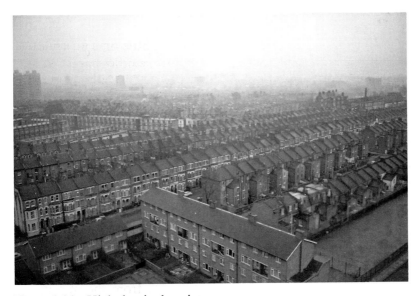

Figure 1.14 High-density housing.

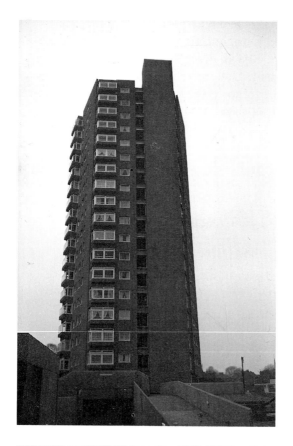

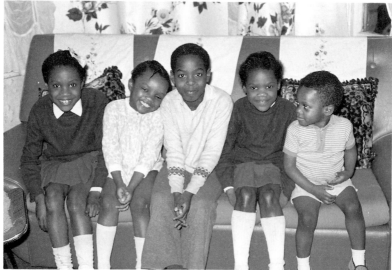

Figure 1.15 High-rise flats and the family who live in one.

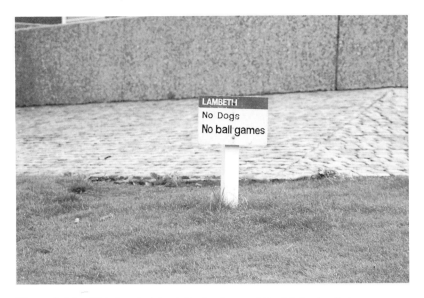

Figure 1.16   This is what is at the bottom of the high-rise flats.

References

1. Court (1976). *Fit for the Future*. Report of Committee on Child Health Services. Comman. 6684 (HMSO)
2. *Health and Personal Social Services Statistics* (1985). (HMSO)
3. Meredith-Davies, J.B. (1983). *Community Health, Preventive Medicine and Social Services*. (London: Baillière Tindall)
4. *Social Trends* (1985). Central Statistical Office, No. 15 (HMSO)
5. General Household Survey (1981). Table 6.15 (HMSO)
6. Townsend, P. and Davidson, N. (1982). *Inequalities in Health*. (Harmondsworth: Penguin)

2

Roles in child care

General practice is a continuing process. The same physician will often care for families for two, three or even four generations over 40 or more years. Except in a few mobile groups the population is stable and static and in Britain less than 1 in 10 families move in a year.

Patients and consultations are rarely 'new'. Most are part of a continuing and long-term care by the same doctor for the same patient in the same family. Care begins from before birth onwards. The mother is seen antenatally and even at pre-conception. The new baby is seen at the children's clinic and then is followed through infancy, childhood, adolescence, parenthood and grandparenthood.

Opportunities are excellent for doctor, mother and child to get to know one another really well.

The average number of consultations per year for each child is six or seven in the first year, three or four in the next 5 years, going down to less than two during adolescence.

In addition to consultations with the doctor, the mother is in regular contact with the health visitors attached to the practice.

In such a continuing system of long-term care, each consultation may be of only 5–10 min. All that is necessary can usually be achieved in this time.

Care for the child begins in the *antenatal* period. The practice antenatal clinic will include the midwife and health visitor attached to the practice and they see the expectant mother, especially primiparae, at each attendance to prepare her for labour and child care (Figure 2.1).

In this context of continuing care dramatic unexpected crises are unusual and general advice and supervision with support and treatment, when necessary, need not take longer than 5–10 min per consultation. Extra time needs to be available for assessments and special occasional difficult multiple problems – usually related to personalities rather than to illness.

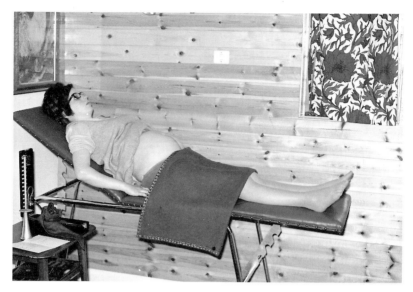

Figure 2.1 Antenatal clinic.

A PLAN FOR CARE

Each doctor and each practice should have a definite plan for child care. The following is one that we have followed.

By doctor

antenatal examinations

first examination when mother and new baby seen during the first 3 weeks of life. Check central neurological system, ears, eyes, hips, testes, height, weight, head circumference.

7 months – doctor checks hearing, vision, gross and fine motor and non-verbal and verbal skills

2 years – check hearing, vision, fine motor, non-verbal skills and, most importantly, language

3 years – as for 2 years

$4\frac{1}{2}$ years – hearing, vision, language, non-verbal skills and co-ordination

By health visitor

during antenatal to get to know mother and family

statutory visit is postnatally

3 months – 1st DPT immunization (or by doctor/nurse)

5 months – 2nd DPT immunization (or by doctor/nurse)

11 months – 3rd DPT immunization (or by doctor/nurse). Also checks mother and baby happy and contented.

13 months – measles immunization (or by doctor/nurse)

18 months – health visitor checks that mother–child relationship going well. Marital and sibling bonds intact, etc. Discussion of child rearing practices and problems, e.g. sleeping, feeding, etc.

Unplanned

In addition to planned consultations mother is free to bring the child at any other time for advice and care.

THE HISTORY

Good history taking is part of every doctor's art. Its worth must never be belittled. Its skills need polishing daily like the front door knob. Facts need to be teased out for accuracy and chronological order. This requires a combination of sensitivity, diplomacy, persistence and mainly patience because the history-giver must not be left with a sense of frustration or of being harried. Family doctors who know the patient and family can pose a few succinct questions that go to the heart of the matter. Hospital paediatricians, on the other hand, will need to ask many more questions before the picture of the child within his family setting becomes clear.

A DIAGNOSIS

Definitive diagnostic labelling is often impossible in real life primary care. Much more important is a *general indicative diagnosis* that should ask questions that must be answered.

Is the child ill or unwell?

What is the likely system involved and what may be the pathology?

Can he/she be treated at home?

If at home, what treatment, supervision and follow-up?

What possible long-term sequelae – emotional, familial or physical?

Should he/she be referred to a specialist?

Is immediate hospital admission necessary?

Reaching a diagnosis in *practice* largely has to be based on history supplemented by examination.

Investigations

Investigations, almost inevitable in hospitals, are less used in general practice. They are unhelpful in the many common conditions of childhood – upper respiratory infections, skin rashes, gastrointestinal upsets and behavioural problems.

They take time, collecting specimens, waiting for results and if blood is taken, they are unpleasant for the child. This does not mean that they are not sometimes necessary for confirmation of specific conditions, such as urinary tract infections, infectious mononucleosis and food poisoning.

The most frequent investigations are urinalysis, full blood counts, throat swab and fecal analyses and most laboratories provide an excellent open access service.

This does not mean that the general practitioner should do no investigations in his practice. Checks for albumin and sugar in urine, dipslide tests for bacteriuria and peak flow measurements of respiratory function and haemoglobin should all be accepted as normal parts of practice.

Hospital admission

If hospital admission is necessary then explain reasons to parents. There should be good reasons for taking this quite significant step:

(1) Is it for the child's good, because parents cannot cope or is it that you, the doctor, are unsure or worried over the condition?

(2) Is it a condition that demands urgent admission, e.g. acute abdomen or respiratory obstruction?

(3) Is it that you, the doctor, feel it all too much for you and you seek to shed the responsibility and the efforts in follow-up?

What should be the content of the doctor's letter?

This differs if referral is for admission or to outpatients. In the former, a concise and logistically correct history with any physical findings is required. It is a good discipline for the GP to put down his own tentative differential diagnosis as this clears his head and, if not good enough, he questions why he is sending the child in the first place. All medication and treatment given should be noted.

In the latter, there is much to be said for the old-fashioned need for a 'specialist' opinion, i.e. the letter goes to a named consultant for a special reason, which is stated in the letter. It will also tell the consultant what the GP hopes to gain from this second opinion and requests an informed reply.

No possible diagnosis

If no diagnosis is possible and there are no reasons for admitting the child to hospital, then follow a routine:

see the child again soon

keep mum busy with the care – feeding or not, keeping notes, giving medicine (if you believe in placebos for symptom relief) – or doing something under your instructions, such as bringing along a sample of urine

inspire confidence, even if you are not that confident yourself

do not engage the family in discussing possibilities of differential diagnoses, especially if some may be serious and dangerous – but inform them of danger signals. If you can't tell what the diagnosis is likely to be, then some parents will think you are not very competent, but with honesty and confidence they can be reassured.

manage the whole nuclear family and get in first before granny starts casting doubts

beware if 'dad comes too'. Ask why he has come. It may indicate anger within the family, or a mother at her 'wits' end'.

When to see again

It is important for continuing care to be organized and arrangements made for a follow-up appointment, or, if this is not considered necessary, then end consultation with 'come again if you are worried'.

Spend time explaining in understandable terms the likely course and outcome of the condition, without undue emphasis on possible complications – but deviations from the expected course should be mentioned as indications for earlier contact.

Repeated requests for unexplained earlier and interim appointments or home visits should alert the doctor and health visitor to give extra support, as it may be an unconscious need for extra attention due to anxiety. Repeated requests signal problems that should be sought out and corrected, if possible. Alternatively, the fault may be the doctor's in misjudging the course and response to care.

All doctors make mistakes and the sooner one learns not only how to live with them but also how to behave towards the patient, the better. This is a hard lesson to learn and much harder for family doctors than hospital doctors because they are likely to go on meeting the mistakes whilst out visiting or shopping. It is, however, necessary for us all to conduct postmortems on mistakes, otherwise one cannot learn from them. It is also a good idea to have a behaviour pattern learned early on in one's career. A short but honest discussion usually pays off better than ignoring the matter. The subject can then be closed.

Family doctors have the advantage over hospital paediatricians in that they know the family. It is knowledge which should be used liberally.

The family doctor (MP) was called by a social worker to a social class 5 one-parent family. The anxious social worker pointed out 'bruises' on the buttocks. The social worker had never seen the father of the child. MP knew him and that he was coloured. A diagnosis of 'Mongolian spots' rather than non-accidental injury was easy (Figure 2.2).

Be big and honest enough to accept the occasional erroneous diagnosis and management of an uncommon condition.

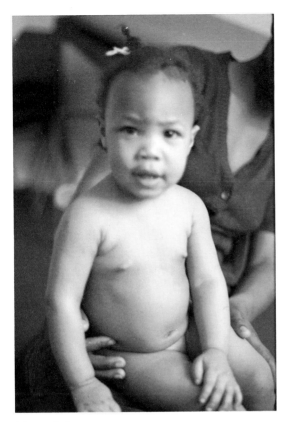

Figure 2.2

Be a personal doctor

Use the consultation, however short it is, as an opportunity for discussing prevention of accidents, smoking, drinking, drugs, education, instruction and reminding mother of previous instructions and preventive care etc. Therefore, good records of child's and family histories, of immunization schedules and adherence, on feeding styles, clothing, behaviour, etc. are important.

Flexibility is an absolute essential. Not all families are like your own and your own family behaviour might not be the best. Therefore, do not judge others by your own standards. Understand and respect each individual and family lifestyle and milieu.

The general practitioner is a *specialist in the common conditions that commonly occur and not in the rarities that rarely happen.*

Be alert to the 'whilst I'm here, doctor' offerings – they may have the answers to indefinite and difficult presentations and situations.

Ask yourself – *'Why have they come?'* Try to understand the parents' thoughts and anticipate their questions and anxieties. These tend to be a part of the local social patterns, but are also influenced by the doctor and how he manages problems, diseases and the practice.

Understand different *parents' estimates and views* of illness and their varying anxiety levels. What may seem minor and trivial to a doctor or nurse may create much anxiety and fear in the mother – often from her own past experiences and what relatives and friends have told her. Such a situation offers special opportunities for reassurance, explanation, education and prevention of future anxieties related to the same minor problem. The reassured mother will be able to cope with it in the future.

SECTION II

Behavioural and Developmental Problems

Together with upper respiratory infections, behavioural and developmental problems are the very stuff of the family doctor's paediatric consultations. It behoves him, therefore, to be knowledgeable in these subjects and to feel confident in dealing with them. In many of the conditions other members of the primary care team have much help to offer.

3

Non-thrivers

'Failure-to-thrive' is usually applied to babies and children in their first 2 years, but some older children also fail to thrive. Most failures-to-thrive are not due to serious underlying diseases. Nevertheless, in the newborn and in the first few weeks of life, there may be a serious, and possibly remediable, cause. Rarities have to be included in the differential diagnosis of common everyday conditions.

Rare causes:
Congenital heart disease
Pyelonephritis and urinary tract abnormalities
Lactose intolerance
Glycogen storage disease

In the UK 98% of births now take place in hospitals. Neonatal examination is carried out in hospital, but mother and child come home within a few days and it is possible for a serious condition to be missed at the initial neonatal examination, or it may not become apparent until after discharge from hospital. The midwife, health visitor and family physician must be alert to such possibilities.

After the postnatal period failure-to-thrive is a problem for the primary care team – it has to be picked up, assessed, diagnosed and managed.

A step-by-step sequence of questions and answers is helpful:

Is there really failure to thrive?

Maternal anxiety may not be supported by the baby's normal and healthy appearance and demeanour. There may be no abnormal physical signs. Frequent serial measures of weight and height plotted on a percentile chart by the health visitor will provide objective data that can be explained to the mother.

The best use of percentile charts is made when height, weight and head circumference are always measured, and differences between them analysed. One measured in isolation is meaningless.

Height	Weight	Head circumference	Condition
All the same percentiles			Average
↓	Normal	Normal	Short stature
Normal	↓	Normal	Failure to thrive
↓	↓	Normal	Chronic illness without mental retardation
↓	↓	↓	CNS deficit

Head Circumference of premature babies

Gestational Age	Weekly increases in cm/week		Total increase in first 16 wks of life
	0–8 wks	9–16 wks	
30–33 weeks WELL	1.1	0.5	13.2 cm
34–37 weeks WELL	0.8	0.4	9.8 cm
30–37 weeks ILL	0.25	0.25	4.0 cm

Despite lack of weight gain, is the baby lively and alert?

This suggests that there is no serious cause. However, note that over-alertness has to be distinguished from irritability of organic disease.

Always relate the child's weight and appearance to those of the parent. A small odd-looking child may have small odd-looking parents.

Never use the term 'funny-looking face' but teach yourself to describe exactly what is seen:

do the eyebrows meet in the middle?
are the epicanthic folds exaggerated?
are the ears low set?
hypoplasia of the jaw, etc.?

In this way one may teach oneself to describe a syndrome.

Is the baby getting enough to eat?

Low birthweight may take 6–12 months to make up and the baby may look 'small for dates' for some months. Probably too little food is still the most likely explanation of non-thriving. Even now with all the health education and training, simple errors can lead to major difficulties.

The middle class mother who equates breast feeding with good motherhood may try desperately to continue breast feeding because of guilt and fear of failure, yet she may have insufficient breast milk for her baby. The young working class mother may find caring for her baby frightening and overwhelming. Confused by advice from friends, mother and mother-in-law she may switch from breast to bottle and back again trying to please everybody, but not her baby.

Premature baby of a 17-year-old single parent, had no fewer than 39 hospital investigations before it was recognized that it was the mother's fear and ignorance that had caused serious underfeeding.

Clinical pointers to type of food deficiency

General caloric deficiency (of all foods) is said chiefly to affect skin and bone.
Major protein deficiency (Kwashiorkor) is characterized by oedema of legs, swollen abdomen and thin sparse hair.

Are other symptoms/signs present?

Repeated vomiting should suggest possible urinary tract infection or pyloric stenosis.
Breathlessness may be due to heart failure or pulmonary infection.

Despite adequate food intake, is there deficient absorption?

Fibrocystic disease is the most common serious absorption defect. Chest infection soon occurs.

Coeliac disease features do not appear until cereals are started.

Intestinal worms can occasionally cause loss of, or failure to gain, weight. However, more often it is surprising how well affected children remain.

Toxoplasmosis and cytomegalovirus infections are rare causes of failure to thrive. Often they are accompanied by convulsions and mental retardation.

Is there a happy family background?

The most likely common factor underlying a baby's failure to thrive is an unhappy family, unhappy mother, unhappy marriage and/or an unhappy baby.

The thin, wan, unhappy, irritable and underweight baby subject to emotional deprivation is one of the most pathetic pictures in paediatrics.

Failure to thrive is a challenge to all who have to care for children. Its causes may be straightforward, but often they pose difficult problems for family and hospital physicians. Take heart from the fact that many babies admitted to hospital because of 'failure to thrive' subsequently gain weight and become healthy babies without any final diagnosis ever being made.

4

Non-eaters

Take note of the following in assessing and managing this very common problem.

history – age, duration, drugs and sex

physical examination – other symptoms

emotional background

HISTORY

Age

Newborn or small baby

Always take seriously. Not taking feeds may be the first sign of disease, e.g. infections and congenital heart diseases.

Toddler

The natural slowing of growth spurt in the second year of life (Figures 4.1 and 4.2) leads to a natural relative lessening of appetite.

Late weaning may mean that the baby is getting a sufficient volume of food from bottle feeds – this may lead to iron deficiency anaemia.

Many normal children when starting to self-feed pat the spoon, dawdle and generally make a fine mess to their own delight but to their parents' impatience and anxiety that not enough food has been consumed (Figure 4.3).

The most likely reason for not eating in toddlers is the normal developmental negative stage dreaded by parents and physicians, but beloved by assertive 2-year-olds. They are quick to notice that refusing

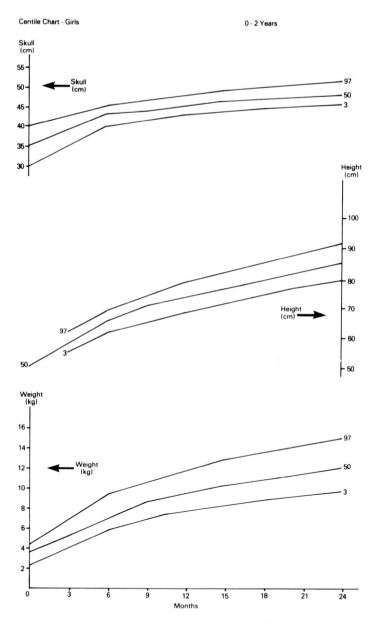

Figure 4.1 Centile chart – girls 0–2 years (from May, *Community Paediatrics*, p. 7, Lancaster: MTP Press, by kind permission).

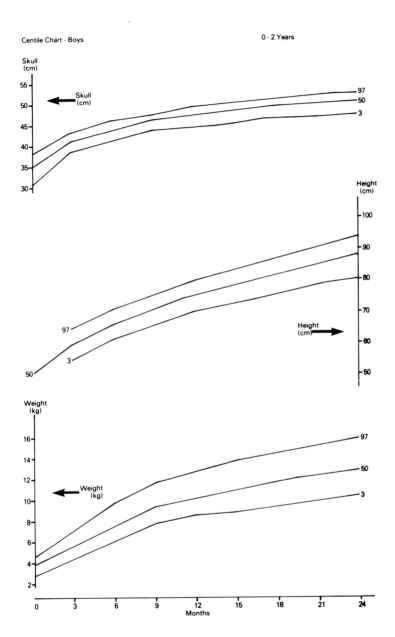

Figure 4.2 Centile chart – boys 0–2 years (from May, *Community Paediatrics*, p. 9, Lancaster: MTP Press, by kind permission).

41

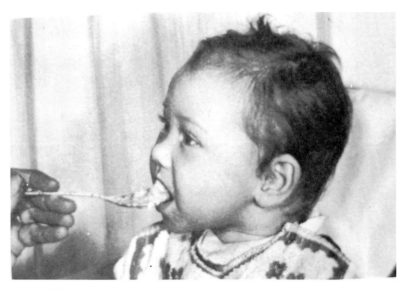

Figure 4.3

food is a good way of raising mum's attention, anxiety and annoyance levels so that mealtimes become battlegrounds, enjoyed by such children.

School child

School takes up a large part of the day and many emotional disturbances at school or at home may cause unhappiness and loss of appetite.

Too many chips, crisps or sweets between meals leave less desire to eat routine dull meals.

Adolescent

Calf love and thinking of the beloved reduce appetite.

Hard drugs can cause anorexia. Anorexia nervosa is another cause of non-eating.

Length of history

A short history of not eating should lead to some concern of possible underlying disorder.

A long history is much more likely to be related to an emotional cause.

Other symptoms and signs

Diarrhoea, vomiting, abdominal pain and malaise suggest a physical cause. Check for possible urinary tract infections, glandular fever, hepatitis and other organic disorders.

Drugs

Iatrogenic anorexia can follow medication with ephedrine and phenytoin.

Sex

Girls are more likely to be concerned with slimming obsessions. Rarely, these may go on to anorexia nervosa. Usually a straightforward discussion with the girl is possible and helpful.

Anorexia nervosa affects girls; boys are only rarely affected. It is accompanied by amenorrhoea, self-induced vomiting, laxative abuse, some facial hirsutism and depression. Pathological toothwear and erosion are frequent[1].

EMOTIONAL FACTORS – APPROACH

Enquire from the mother how much she thinks the child should eat and drink. Discuss with the mother the wide variations of appetite in normal children, not only between children but from day to day in the same child. Variations in appetites and tastes, likes and dislikes for certain foods may have physiological bases related to the body's needs.

Work out planned strategies with the mother to make mealtimes pleasurable:

no fuss if food is left
recognize and understand food fads
offer choice of foods on occasions

Why is the mother so worried about the child's eating patterns? Is she trying to produce a large child like her friends and the baby next door? Are grandmothers pressurizing with comments and advice? Is there a problem of mother/child relationship? Are there other features of this whenever they come together – at bed time, toileting, shopping, visiting, taking to school, etc.?

If the mother remains not reassured and unconvinced of the normality of the situation then:

chart weight on a percentile chart over weeks/months (this gives everyone a respite)

ask mother to write down everything that child eats and drinks over a week or longer.

Both these actions, hopefully, will provide factual evidence that all is well.

If not, a referral to a known local paediatrician is a good therapeutic action – but the referral letter must state the reasons and background with the hope that he/she will reassure the mother. Even better, a preliminary telephone call to the paediatrician will be effective.

James F. age 2½
'He don't eat a thing!'
He stands like a defiant cherub, a picture of good health (Figure 4.4)

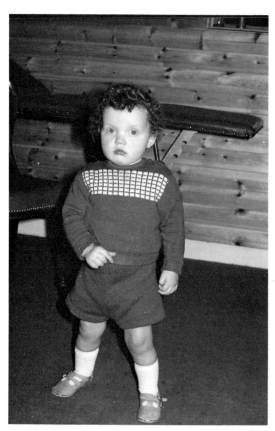

Figure 4.4

James was born when Mum was 42.

A Roman Catholic, she was unhappy with this, her fifth pregnancy. She could not consider a termination of her pregnancy.

The pregnancy was uneventful.

James is adored, the 'pet of the family'.

Mother feels guilty in not wanting him originally.

She gives in to every whim, feeds him delicacies and left-over titbits.

James, with his ginger curls, dressed in his Mum's best knitting, finds the mealtime battles most enjoyable.

Mum presents the child as 'her illness' and needs sympathetic insight and explanation of the emotional mechanisms of James' behaviour.

Reference

1. Smith, B.G.N. and Knight, J.K. (1984). A comparison of patterns of tooth wear with aetiological factors. *Br. Dent. J.*, **157,** 16–19

5

Non-sleepers

Assuming that illness can be excluded, then non-sleeping requires a careful and patient analysis of parental background, personality and beliefs.

Does non-sleeping really matter? Not very much to the child, but very much to parents. They suffer because of lack of sleep and worry that their child may not be normal, like their friends' children.

Children have differing requirements for amounts of sleep, just as adults. They develop different patterns and habits of sleep. Some like to sleep more in the day and want to play in the middle of the night. It is difficult for parents to accept that it takes some children time to accept that night-time is for sleeping.

Some mentally retarded children have a sleep reversal in the second year of life.

Once the habit of non-sleeping is developed it is difficult to break. Bedtime must be made pleasant. This is difficult when Mum has other jobs waiting for her and when Dad is waiting for his evening meal.

When the child wakes at night he should be kept in bed with minimal handling but reassuring comforting. Taking him into the parental bed should be resisted for as long as possible because once established the habit is difficult to break and may disrupt the marriage. Often it is part of a stressed parent–child relationship accompanying other behavioural symptoms when parents and child come together, e.g. mealtimes, or excessive clinging and school problems in older children.

Nevertheless, a liberal flexible approach is essential. Some parents find that peaceful nights can only be achieved if the non-sleeper is allowed into their bed. They should not be made to feel guilty as failures. Eventually the habit will cease with parents and child none the worse for the experience. Strict separation of children from parents at night is a relatively recent custom in man's history.

Be prepared for the unusual.

Sandra B. a very pretty 7-year-old was afraid to fall asleep. Sandra normally slept with her mother. Sandra's mother was a prostitute who sometimes brought her customers home into the shared bed. Sandra was very upset to be removed.

Two couples (well known to the practice) regularly 'wife-swapped'. Adam K. liked to stay awake and to go into the parental bedroom to 'see who Mummy had in bed with her!'

What about sleeping medicines?

If possible do without, but commonsense must prevail and sometimes it may be best to try and break the vicious circle with a mild hypnotic.

6

Crying babies

Crying is the first communication which the baby makes. Normal babies cry more quickly after a stimulus than retarded babies. Premature babies have a feeble cry.

The early cry, from a nasty stimulus, is short and staccato, rising to a crescendo. If the stimulus is repeated, this leads to another crescendo, so the cry seems to be repetitive.

In an older baby, the duration of the cry is longer but rhythmic so it seems much slower and more urgent.

Later still the cry has more pitch, syllables and more variety, making it sound more plaintive and meaningful.

Some conditions have special cries. The cry of cerebral irritation, e.g. kernicterus or meningitis, is shrill and *high pitched*. A cretin, or baby with hypothyroidism, has a *hoarse, gruff cry*. A *cat-like cry* is said to be heard in cri-du-chat syndrome (mental retardation microcephaly, low set ears, usually seen in females, due to a partial deletion of the short arm of chromosome 5).

Crying has to be differentiated from *stridor* which is essentially an inspiratory noise. Very ill children *whimper*, but a child with severe otitis media, for example, may *scream* with pain. The subjects of child abuse also cry a great deal, due to unhappiness.

Babies aged 6–9 months are particularly liable to cry if a stranger suddenly appears and sometimes if their parents appear in strange places. Also, they may cry if a stranger appears impassive, so it is a very good idea to talk to the mother.

Older children sometimes cry at every disappointment. This may be a sign of lack of confidence.

Mothers claim that they recognize the cry of their newborn baby long before the father does so.

Crying of young babies is purposeful – it may be brought on by anoxia, pain, hunger and sometimes contentment!

7

Late walkers

'Walking' means walking alone and unaided. Variations are wide but between 12–17 months should be considered normal. Illingworth's remark that *late walking* is **not** an orthopaedic problem is very wise[1]. In a child aged 18 months who is not yet walking, the following sequence of questions need answering.

ARE OTHER MOTOR MILESTONES NORMAL?

Did he roll over by 8 months?

Sit alone by 9 months? (Figure 7.1)

Pull to stand by 13 months?

If so, reassurance is almost certainly in order. If not, then seek causes.

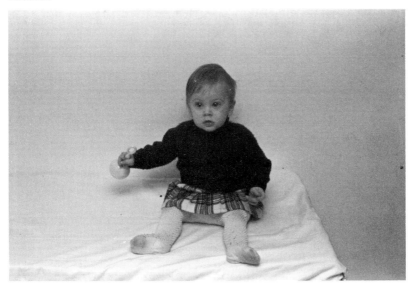

Figure 7.1

WHAT WAS THE CHILD'S EARLY METHOD OF PROGRESSION?

Did he creep before crawling and late, (e.g. 13 months)? (Figure 7.2)

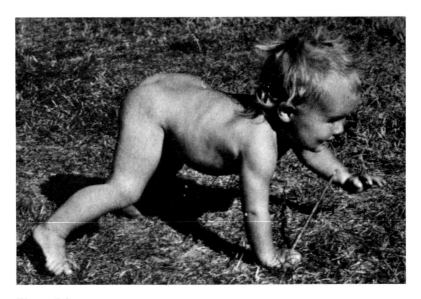

Figure 7.2

Did he never crawl but shuffled on his bottom and that late (e.g. 12–16 months)?

Then he will walk late[2] (e.g. 18–28 months). Mother can then be reassured (both creeping and shuffling are familial habits).

IF THE MOTOR MILESTONES ARE DELAYED, ARE OTHER MILESTONES ALSO DELAYED?

If so, then *general developmental delay* is present. This may be due to:

lack of opportunity (see story of Josie, p. 59)

mental retardation – in which case other parameters of development (e.g. non-verbal, verbal and social) will be even more delayed than the motor development

sensory loss – severe degrees of both hearing and visual loss cause verbal and other developmental skills to be late

cerebral palsy with mental retardation – in this case the motor development and examination will be *abnormal* as well as delayed with varying degrees of mental delay.

EXAMINATION OF MOTOR DEVELOPMENT WHEN MOTOR MILESTONES ARE DELAYED

This requires an assessment of:

muscle power and tone

reflexes

the continued presence of some primitive reflexes and the absence of others

symmetry of reaction.

Muscle tone and power

This is a very difficult examination to undertake and interpret and experience is probably the only reliable method of interpretation of any but extreme variations. Furthermore, the opportunity for family doctors to become experienced is limited. One of the best ways is to use the regular first examination of a *newborn baby*.

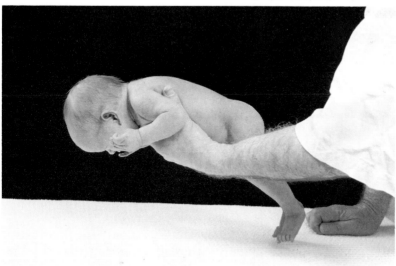

Figure 7.3 Testing muscle tone in the newborn (from O'Doherty, *Neurological Examination of the Newborn*, p. 96, Lancaster: MTP Press, by kind permission).

Hold the baby's abdomen in the palm of one hand and bob first the feet and then the hands up and down with the other. It only takes a moment to do, it will give few, if any, dividends at the time, but it will allow the doctor, one day, to recognize a difference from normal and, thus, not to miss the case of cerebral palsy, which a practice will have once every 12–14 years.

For the *18-month-old* who presents as a non-walker, the best way to examine him is for the doctor to kneel on the floor, the baby sitting on the doctor's lap, looking at his mother (Figure 7.4). In this way, the baby will be happily relaxed and reflexes are easy to test, the tendon hammer coming from behind.

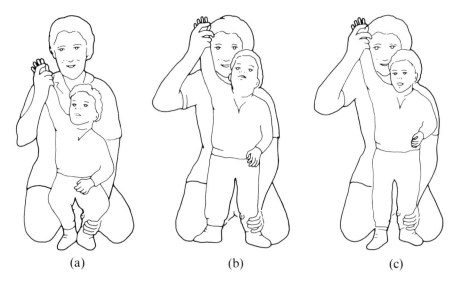

(a)   (b)   (c)

Figure 7.4   Testing muscle tone in a child: (a) hold ankle and pull on opposite arm; (b) if patient has good tone he can extend held leg and (c) take a step forward. Repeat for opposite side – should be symmetrical.

A good way to test the power in the lower limbs is to have the baby on the lap, as described. Put one foot of the baby firmly on the ground and hold it there. The doctor's other hand pulls the baby's contralateral arm upwards. If tone in the quadriceps is good, the muscle will contract and the baby rises to the standing position. When power and tone are poor, the baby only flops forward. Repeat for the other side and particularly note any asymmetry. If hypotonia is present there is usually a history of previous hypotonia, e.g. late head holding, late sitting, whilst poor power will usually have a history of previous weakness, i.e. swallowing and respiratory difficulties.

Unusual exceptions are muscle dystrophies which are progressive (e.g. Duchenne) which may not present until 2–3 years of age.

Not only is the diagnosis of altered tone difficult, but one of the great pitfalls in the diagnosis of cerebral palsy, especially the diplegic type, is that initial hypotonia is replaced by hypertonia, the change usually taking place between 12 and 20 months.

Reflexes

An easy way to elicit reflexes in babies is by holding them as described above. Although easy to elicit, if present, they are difficult to interpret as children differ in response, but there should be no difference between the response on one side of the body from the other. If this is suspected, listing to one side and lack of movement on the same side should be looked for.

The palmar grasp reflex

This usually disappears by 2–3 months. A finger or pencil put in the baby's palm from the ulnar side will produce strong finger flexion (Figure 7.5)

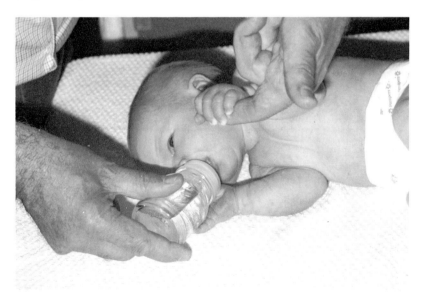

Figure 7.5 Automatic palmar grasp in the newborn (from O'Doherty, *Neurological Examination of the Newborn*, p. 14, Lancaster: MTP Press, by kind permission).

The Moro reflex

Cradle the baby's head in the palm of one hand and lie the baby along the other hand and forearm, supporting the upper trunk and shoulders. Allow the head to drop a few cms. by lowering the cradling hand. Catch the dropped head (Figure 7.6).

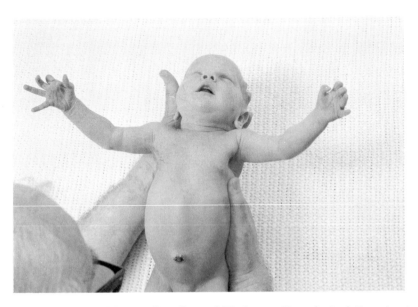

Figure 7.6 The Moro reflex (from O'Doherty, *Neurological Examination of the Newborn*, p. 123, Lancaster: MTP Press, by kind permission).

A normal response is symmetrical extension and abduction of the arms, with spreading of the fingers followed by flexion of the arms, as in an embrace. Usually, the legs flex. The Moro reflex is present at birth and usually disappears by 8–12 weeks.

Abnormalities

May be asymmetric (reproducible) in hemiplegia.

May persist beyond time in cerebral palsy.

May be extremely easy to produce in hyperactivity, neurological damage and immaturity.

The asymmetrical tonic neck reflex

This reflex usually disappears by 3–5 months. It is also known as the 'fencing' or 'roman gladiator position'. When the head is turned to one side the arm on that side extends whilst the other flexes towards the occiput (Figure 7.7). A similar but weaker reaction is seen in the legs.

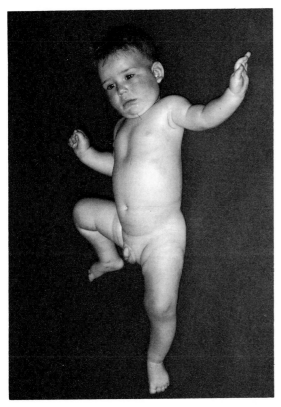

Figure 7.7 Asymmetrical tonic neck response (from O'Doherty, *Neurological Examination of the Newborn*, p. 165, Lancaster: MTP Press, by kind permission).

These reflexes may all persist beyond the normal times in cerebral palsy and they should be tested in all cases of motor delay.

Downwards and sideways parachute reflexes

These are normal in children as they learn to balance. They may be absent or markedly delayed in cerebral palsy.

Asymmetry

As already mentioned, this is an important finding and affects movement, power and tone as well as reflexes (Figure 7.8).

The hemiplegia of cerebral palsy is usually the least serious type of cerebral palsy and the arm appears more affected than the leg.

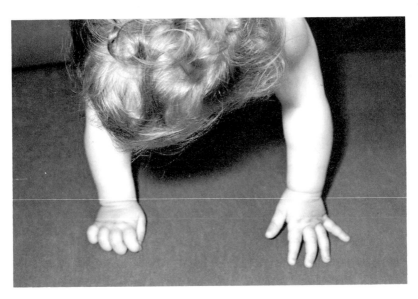

Figure 7.8 Forwards parachute response asymmetrical (from O'Doherty, *Neurological Examination of the Newborn*, p. 174, Lancaster: MTP Press, by kind permission).

INTERPRETATIONS

A child with ONLY a motor problem, hypotonia and sluggish reflexes will have *benign hypotonia* or rarely, *lower motor muscle disease*, such as congenital neuropathies, dystrophia myotonia or progressive muscular dystrophy.

A few of these children with *benign hypotonia* will be found clumsy at school later[3].

A child with hypertonia and brisk reflexes is likely to have a *spastic type of cerebral palsy*.

A child with hypotonia, brisk jerks and residual primitive reflexes may have an *athetoid type of cerebral palsy*.

A child with hypotonia, unsteady gait and brisk reflexes is most likely to have a *cerebellar problem*.

A change in tone in some types of cerebral palsy already described may occur over a time.

ILLUSTRATIVE CASE

This case illustrates a delayed motor development due to environment.

Josie was admitted to hospital with a chest infection. When better, she was noted, at 2½ years of age, not to be walking. She was thoroughly examined and no abnormality was discovered. She could pull to stand and stand. With the help of the physiotherapist, she was soon persuaded to walk. But walk alone she would not. Even holding someone's fifth finger was enough, but she would *not* walk unaided. Whilst her medical attendant was thinking up ways to achieve independence, Josie found the solution herself. She walked along 'holding on' to her dress (Figure 7.9). This gave her enough confidence to manage.

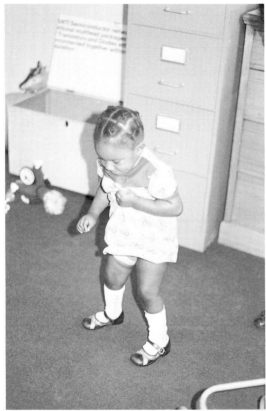

Figure 7.9

Josie, who was born in Nigeria, was fostered by a Caucasian woman who was unregistered. She fostered several other children as well, and on questioning her, it became apparent that Josie spent most of the day standing in her cot without the opportunity of learning to walk.

References

1. Illingworth, R. S. (1975). *Common Diseases of Childhood.* (Edinburgh: Churchill Livingstone)
2. Robson, P. (1970). Shuffling, hitching, scooting or sliding. Some observations in 30 otherwise normal children. *Develop. Med. Child. Neurol.*, **12**, 608–17
3. Drillien, C. M. (1964). Correlation between pre-school testing and I.Q. testing in school. In *Growth and Development of the Prematurely Born Infant*, p. 20 (Edinburgh: Churchill Livingstone)

8

Late talkers

REQUIREMENTS FOR SPEECH AND LANGUAGE

Adequate hearing

Someone to whom one can listen and learn

Adequate thought processes and perceptive powers

Adequate organization and production of motor skills (100 muscles needed to say a word)

Someone to listen – an audience to talk with

NORMAL DEVELOPMENT

Names a few life-size objects by 16 months

Names miniature toys by 24 months

Can relate to two objects by $2\frac{1}{2}$ years

Knows big and small by 3 years

Knows colours and prepositions by 4 years

DEFINITION OF LATE TALKERS

Not responding to name or 'no' at 1 year

No distinct word at 18 months

No sentences of three words by 3 years. Only 10% of speech unintelligible

TYPES OF SPEECH DEFECTS

Simple developmental language delay

comprehension of language satisfactory

central or 'inner' language normal (intellectual coding, decoding and integration)

limited vocabulary which may be clearly understood or difficult to understand

due to a developmental lag or poor environmental stimulation, no one to listen or talk with

prognosis good

More severe expressive aphasia

comprehension of language satisfactory

central coding system normal or mildly delayed

dyspraxia – unintelligible speech of varying degrees

often other developmental immaturities, e.g. eneuresis, clumsiness

common in cerebral palsy

more common in boys

prognosis depends upon receiving adequate expert help in preschool time

can be due to environmental deprivation

Receptive aphasia

delayed comprehension

central language delayed

expressive language may be almost normal in content and intelligibility

diagnosis may be:

Mental retardation

This is the most common cause. Non-verbal skills are also delayed.

Deafness

Hearing is deficient. Other forms of communication, e.g. gesturing, eye contact and touching are present.

Specific language disorder

The child is not deaf. Non-verbal skills are normal. There is often echolalia. The child 'cannot seem to make sense of his social environment'. He may have ritualistic, compulsive behaviour; severe degrees may be diagnosed as autistic (especially if seen in psychiatric clinic!).

All three types need expert help with diagnosis and treatment.

WHAT CAN THE GP DO?

He should know that delay is *never* due to 'tongue tie' or 'laziness'. He should take a history of *language environment*.

is there someone who regularly and constantly talks to the child and listens to him?

what is the language of the parents like?

has there been a succession of au pairs, etc. speaking different languages?

is the child at a busy nursery or at a child-minder with little individual attention?

Delayed speech is only a symptom. As in any other medical problem, try and make a diagnosis.

HOW TO MAKE A DIAGNOSIS

Risk factors

Speech delay is more common in prematurity; breech and forceps deliveries; low birth weight of less than 2500 g; mother aged less than 18 years; high parity; and/or one parent is of low IQ.

Diagnosis of child's linguistic skills

Comprehension, central and expressive speech must be measured, otherwise no differential diagnosis can be made.

Hearing must be tested

High frequency nerve deafness may be missed as speech is often more distorted than severely delayed. Low frequency conductive deafness is more often due to middle ear deafness.

Measurement of social and non-verbal skills is essential

If these are poor, mental retardation or, rarely, autism are likely diagnoses. Mental retardation is the most frequent cause of delayed speech. It is also an important diagnosis to make.

Deprivational speech delay

This will have been suspected from the history. Another type of deprivational delay may be due to a depressed mother'. She may reflect an absence of 'an audience to listen to verbalization'. Starte[1] found almost *all* the two-year-olds with poor language development had associated family problems, often maternal depression.

It is very difficult to make the differential diagnosis between *deafness* and *specific language delay* in some cases as the child with the latter will not attend to sounds, so one does not know whether he *cannot* or *will not* listen. Sometimes crossed acoustic reflexes brain stem response tests have to be undertaken in order to make the diagnosis.

The *differential diagnosis between deafness and mental retardation* is also difficult in some cases. Firstly, because both may be present and, secondly, because mentally retarded children may not motivate well to hearing tests which involve their co-operation. It is best, therefore, to use one of the newer tests available which do not need the child's co-operation.

Remember, if the *expressive language is affected*, to look for clumsiness (these children have a history of poor educational skills) and mild types of cerebral palsy.

HOW TO TREAT

If there is simple developmental delay, then simple treatment will suffice. Reassure the parents and impress upon them that they are the child's best therapists. Explain how they can best teach the child to talk and review the child in 3 months' time. The health visitor could be involved. (See Appendix.)

Do not assume that simply by sending the child to a nursery or playgroup that this will help the child's language. Children learn to speak from adults, not from each other. More adult speech is heard at home than at an average nursery.

If diagnosis is receptive or expressive aphasia, mental retardation or deafness, etc. refer to a Child Development Centre for full assessment and diagnosis. Some Centres offer treatment, others refer on to suitable units.

IS TREATMENT WORTHWHILE?

The National Child Development Survey found that 10-13% of 7-year-olds had defective speech and the majority of these (56%) did badly in school at 11 years[2].

On the other hand, a study in America of children who had expert preschool help found they had done better in many ways by the age of 20 years, compared with a control group who had had no such help[3].

To be meaningful, diagnosis must be precise and help must be expert. In these cases, treatment IS worthwhile.

ILLUSTRATIVE CASE

Gerald was non-verbal at 2 years 8 months. He was referred to the Child Development Centre by his family doctor as a behaviour problem. Gerald had two fixations – he loved to play with water and he loved furry material.

A developmental examination revealed that his motor and non-verbal skills were age appropriate. He was immature socially, although his personal toileting and eating skills, etc. were normal. His language was examined in detail. He understood language to an 18-month level. He was unable to symbolize miniature toys, showing no understanding of their use. He was not quite non-verbal, but his words were inappropriate. For example, when shown a picture of a flower (not a rose) he said 'ring – a, ring a'. Echolalia was marked – 'Show me the shoes'. Gerald – 'shoes, shoes'. His hearing was difficult to test, he did not appear to respond to conventional testing, or only erratically. A crossed acoustic reflex test (done by the Centre's audiologist on a computerized test as an out-patient) showed the presence of adequate hearing. Vision was satisfactory. Although his non-verbal skills were age appropriate, Gerald loved to line up the toy cars, or any other toy, and was upset if the line was altered. His love of furry material had led his mother to make him a waistcoat of furry material and in

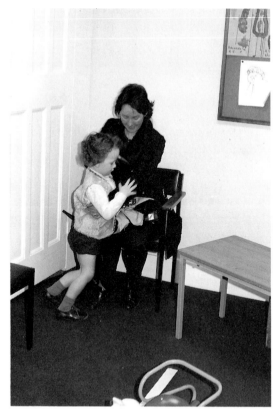

Figure 8.1

Figure 8.1 he is seen wearing it and licking the fur collar on his mother's overcoat.

A diagnosis of specific language disorder with some autistic features was made. Gerald was intensively tested and treated by the Centre's speech therapist, and he attended the special nursery for language-impaired children. He made some improvement, particularly as the psychologist helped his two fixations with behaviour modification. He was not able to attend normal school at five, and went to a Language Unit. By age eight, however, he was able to attend normal school. He has some learning problems, but is coping. Although his reading is age appropriate, he does not understand what he reads. Spelling is $2\frac{1}{2}$ years behind chronological age and socialization is poor.

References

1. Starte, G. D. (1978). The poor communicating two-year-old and his family. *J. R. Coll. Gen. Pract.*, **4,** 880
2. Butler, N. R., Peckham, C. S. and Sheridan, M. (1973). Speech defects in children aged 7 years. *Br. Med. J.*, **1,** 253
3. Epstein, A. S. and Weikart, D. P. (1980). *The Longitudinal Follow-up of the Ypsilante-Carnegie Infant Education Project*. (High/Scope Press) (from Children's Bureau)

9

The overactive child

There is considerable confusion over the overactive child. There are two reasons for this, firstly, because hyperactivity and clumsiness are often thought of as synonymous, which they are not, although both can be present in the same child; and secondly, there is no general agreement about whether the *'minimal brain damage syndrome'* exists and, if so, how frequently it occurs.

'Hyperactivity' is thought to be present in 4–10% of American children under 12 years of age[1], whilst under 1% of children in the UK will have this diagnosis[2]. The best way is to note the age of the child.

IF THE CHILD IS AGED 2–4 YEARS

He is almost certainly male and his activity should be studied.

(a) Is he really *not* hyperactive, but flitting purposelessly from one thing to another? Give him two or three constructive toys to play with. Does he play meaningfully with them or not? This is an excellent test.

(b) Is he really just determined to defy authority at all costs, be it mother or his medical attendant?

(c) Is he pleasantly naughty with a parent who is completely at his mercy, having no idea of discipline?

(d) Does he also have a history of late toilet training, poor and indistinct speech?

If the case fits (a) he is probably *mentally retarded or severely deprived* (or both).

If (b), the diagnosis is probably an extreme example of the *defiant, negative* 2–3-year-old.

If (c), there is a *mother/child relationship problem*. Look for problems at other times when mother and child are together, e.g. feeding, bedtime, etc.

If (d), he probably really is *hyperactive with an exhausted mother*. A 'low' stimulus atmosphere helps and play with one thing at a time with a calm parent, etc. Nursery school probably does not help this type of child.

The prognosis for (b) and (c) is good, and (d) is likely to 'grow out of it'.

IF THE CHILD IS OF SCHOOL AGE

Here the diagnosis is much more difficult and needs fairly expert differential diagnosis. Many children are missed, many are referred to Child Guidance clinics and many just lag behind at school work and are thought to be 'lazy'. Useful categories are as follows.

Minimal cerebral dysfunction syndrome

This is characterized by a scatter of 'soft' neurological signs, e.g. hypertonia, restlessness, vestibular, proprioceptive, visual and frequently spatial inaptitudes, agnosia and apraxia.

True 'clumsy' syndrome

These children, usually boys, have a long history of being clumsy. They only reach clinical observation when they are in educational difficulties. They are used to failing at physical problems, they have poor body image and when tested on standard tests of motor impairment (e.g. Stott test) will be three standard deviations below their age expectancy, at least. Gross motor function is usually more affected than fine motor control.

Stott Test of Motor Impairment measures degrees of impairment against normal attainments for age. Five sub-headings are gross motor, balance, eye-motor co-ordination, fine manipulation and simultaneous movements.

Missed mental retardation

The retardation is unlikely to be severe, but such children are characterized by 'useless' activity, with short concentration and attention spans. Also, these children have low school achievements.

Clumsy but with learning problems

Type 2 children usually have difficulties with handwriting, but some clumsy children, as defined above, have severe difficulties with reading and spelling as well. On the 'Pollak Tapper', a simple device which shows up difficulties in visual and auditory sequencing[3], these children are shown to have visual sequencing and memory problems, auditory sequencing usually being normal (Figure 9.1).

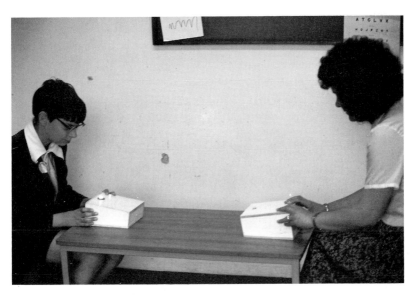

Figure 9.1   The Pollak Tapper.

Conduct disorder with aggressive overactivity

These children are usually diagnosed as 'clumsy' or 'overactive' in retrospect. They are often anxious children with environmental and emotional deprivation. Learning difficulties are a frequent accompaniment. They come to attention because of stealing, vandalism or truancy. They are rather solitary children and tend to be aggressive towards society.

MANAGEMENT

All these five types of overactive children can be helped by expert therapists working on each child's particular problems and can produce considerable improvements in their motor deficits. Moreover, this improvement can be sustained over time. Weekly therapy, firstly alone, later in small groups, over a 6 month period is much more effective than concentrated daily sessions over a short period of a month.

Not only do the children achieve motor, hand-eye and sensory improvement, but they begin to gain confidence. These children are characterized by their acceptance of failure, they often have a high achieving sibling with whom their parents constantly compare them unfavourably, but when they see they can begin to achieve, their confidence becomes much improved. They begin to attempt physical tasks, unafraid of the expected ridicule and this also spins off to other areas. School work improves.

An experienced occupational therapist is another most useful member of the team in helping children with spatial and orientation problems. Remedial teachers who understand the exact nature of the child's problem can help with reading, spelling and writing. These two workers are particularly helpful for type 4 children (clumsy with learning problems).

Type 5 children (conduct disorder with aggressive hyperactivity) need expert psychiatric care. Nevertheless, if they have much motor incoordination, physiotherapy can help by improving motor skills. The individual attention often helps their low self-image, so characteristic of these children.

References

1. Stephenson, P.S. (1975). The hyperkinetic child, some misleading assumptions. *Canad. Med. Assoc. J.*, **113,** 764
2. Rutter, M., Tizard, J. and Whitmore, K. (1970). *Education, Health and Behaviour.* (London: Longmans)
3. Pollak, M. and Tuchler, H. (1982). The Pollak Tapper. *Headteachers' Review*, summer

10

School problems

Children from the age of 5 to leaving school at 16–18 years will spend about 20% of their lives at school (and another 33% sleeping!) School and its activities thus play an important part in an important time of their development.

The problems that school children may experience are of two types – those *due to* school and those that occur *at school* (Figure 10.1).

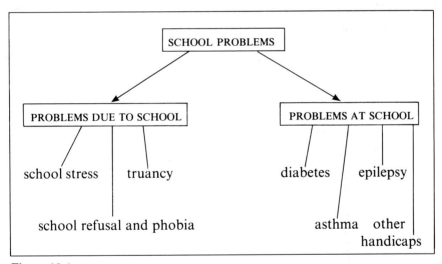

Figure 10.1

From the National Child Development Study[1] the following are the numbers of problems and medical disorders that may be expected in schoolchildren (5–16) in a general practice of 2500 persons.

50 children will need to wear glasses by the age of 11 (just over half of these will have a history of squint).

But one-half of those who should be wearing glasses will not be doing so.

20 children will absent from school – 7 without a proper reason.

10 will be poor readers.

9 (2 primary and 7 secondary) will have gone to school without breakfast.

7 will be receiving special education.

6 will have serious educational problems.

3 will be uneducable.

1 will never learn to read or write.

Medical problems

35 children will be *obese* (20% or more overweight) – more likely in girls and in social classes 4 and 5 (Figure 10.2).

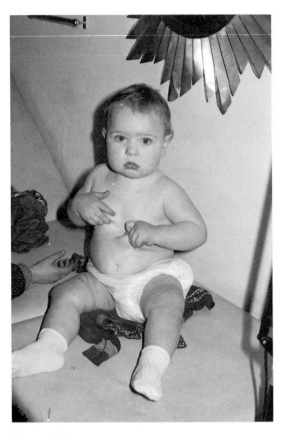

Figure 10.2

39 wet their beds – more in social classes 4 and 5 and where there are bad parental relationships.

19 suffer from eczema.

18 suffer from asthma.

18 suffer from otitis media.

PROBLEMS ARISING FROM SCHOOL

School stress syndrome

The child presents to his family doctor with psychosomatic symptoms, such as headache, abdominal pains, or other reasons for being away from school.

A sensitive history will reveal that the symptoms occur on school day mornings or, conversely, are absent at weekends and holidays. Further enquiry shows that the child is 'trailing' at school and is often in the 'remedial' group. Dislike of school is not usually directly stated. The aetiology is a triad of ambitious parents, a competitive school class and a child with an IQ in the lower range of normal, e.g. 75–85.

This situation calls for a close liaison between parents, family doctor, teachers and educational psychologist. This rarely happens. This is a pity because the family doctor has much to offer. He knows the child, the parents and the family background and he can bring some of his highest skills to the situation. Counselling parents and child successfully, alleviating the problem for the child without hurting the parents needs delicate, sensitive handling. The school doctor and the psychologist may advise a change of school and this may be the solution. Just treating the initial symptom is merely papering over the cracks.

School refusal or school phobia

This is a different problem from the school stress syndrome, although psychosomatic symptoms are a frequent accompaniment. It is a serious condition, requiring expert help and the prognosis is often poor. The phobia is not related to school but rather a fear of leaving home. The onset is usually sudden, the child having previously been a good school attender. The two sexes are equally affected within the range of 8–12 years. The child is conscientious with conforming parents.

School phobia is a childhood neurosis triggered off by a family problem, e.g. marital discord, divorce, bereavement, an accident or serious illness. It is wise to seek psychiatric help early because both parents and child need help. If the child is particularly anxious, short-term tranquillizer therapy may be useful, and if the anxiety of the parents cannot be reduced, a temporary attendance of the child at a psychiatric day centre for children may be advisable. The time for return to school is a decision demanding careful consideration involving the school and the class teacher as well as psychiatrist and psychologist.

A change of school is not advisable, although parents will often request it. It represents an attempt to unload anxiety by blaming the school and will not help the child.

School truancy

The prevalence of school truancy is difficult to estimate. Reynolds, studying nine secondary schools in South Wales, found rates varying from 11 to 33% of the school population[2]. Rutter found numbers of 'very poor attenders' differed not only between schools in the same area of Inner London, but also between children at primary schools and secondary schools (the latter being higher)[3]. This study found rates ranging from 6 to 26%. Truants differ from school phobics or refusers in several ways. The onset is usually insidious, with a previous poor attendance record. The children are usually younger than those refusing school.

Truancy is a childhood conduct disorder. Truants have histories of being disruptive when they do attend school and are rebellious against authority in general. Very often they are both socially and emotionally deprived. Many, but not all, have IQs towards the lower end of average.

Unlike school phobia, truancy rarely arises from a family crisis but is caused by parental lack of interest in the child's development and school achievement. There is a close relationship between social deprivation and poor school attendance. Rutter analysed 'poor attenders' and found that school attendances were particularly poor on Mondays and Fridays, often for very trivial reasons such as parents getting late out of bed or a general lack of importance for getting the child to attend school.

Treatment depends upon how well the whole family situation can be helped. The success or failure of outcome is therefore highly dependent upon the calibre of the parents. With regard to the truancy itself, a firm and energetic return to school is required, backed by close liaison between the family, teachers and school welfare officers. This is essential so that any further lapse can be dealt with at once. If the child, in addition, has a learning problem, this needs special remedial help because improvement increases the child's motivation to go to school.

The family doctor and the primary care team with considerable knowledge of the whole family can promote good child rearing practices to parents when he sees them for other reasons.

Social deprivation, emotional neglect and lack of parenting skills produce different effects in babies and children at different times in their lives. During school age truancy may be one, and juvenile delinquency another.

An at-risk register of families suffering from social disadvantages will enable the primary care team to offer special care to these parents when the children are young, helping them to understand their children's developing needs, the importance of learning how to learn, and to take an interest in their school progress.

ILLNESSES WHICH THE CHILD TAKES TO SCHOOL

For the school, chronic illness is more important than acute episodic illnesses because the child has to try and adjust his illness to his school day.

Diabetes

A general practice of 2000 patients can expect to have one or two diabetic patients under the age of 15 years. Diabetes in children often has a dramatic acute onset and sometimes children can be controlled at hospital and returned to school without the school doctor and/or nurse being informed.

James, aged eight, was overweight and lethargic. He suddenly lost weight and was found to have glycosuria. Initial control of his diabetes was undertaken in hospital and James was soon back at school. Neither the hospital nor family doctor informed the school medical services of the diagnosis. Soon James had times at school when he was tired, irritable, inattentive and restless. One weekend, he had such an attack and the family doctor was called. The doctor, having the advantage of knowing about James' diabetes, was able to diagnose his hypoglycaemic attacks.

It is important for the school to know about a diabetic child so that school meals can be suitable. Their timing may need adjusting – for example to include a mid-morning snack. It is also necessary for the school nurse or doctor to know if the child is going to have a very heavy sports day and may, thus, require less insulin. The necessity to test visual acuity frequently must be remembered.

M.P., an adolescent boy, was brought into a hospital casualty department in a comatose state. The clue to his diagnosis was his immaculate white cricket clothes. A card saying that he was a diabetic was found in his pocket. His hypoglycaemic attack was rapidly treated. Not one of the accompanying cricketers knew that he was a diabetic.

Asthma

As many as 25% of children experience wheezing attacks[4]. Although not all wheezers are asthmatics, asthma is common in schoolchildren and the school needs to be informed whether the child has a prophylactic or therapeutic inhaler. The class teacher needs to know how this works and, in particular, how often (or seldom) and how many puffs the child requires.

Acute emotional stress or sudden physical exercise are factors that can trigger an acute attack at school. It is important that school teachers should know how to cope with acute asthmatic attacks and not immediately send the child to the accident–emergency department of the local hospital. His GP may have spent considerable efforts to 'defuse' the family from going straight to the hospital.

The aim should be to encourage the asthmatic child to lead a normal school life within his limits. This requires collaboration between parents, family doctor, school and the school health services.

Epilepsy

A group practice will have at least one schoolchild with troublesome epilepsy. Holdsworth and Whitmore found that only one third of epileptic children in normal schools were making satisfactory progress, one half were below average standards, and one sixth had serious behaviour problems[5].

If the epileptic child *is doing well at school*, the school doctor and teachers need to know:

What is his drug treatment?

Does he take it?

Does he need to take it in school time?

Do the parents ensure that supplies of drugs are available? (The most likely cause of a convulsion is not taking the drugs regularly.)

How to deal with a major seizure if it occurs at school.

How does the family and the child cope with the problem, especially keeping the child at school regularly, and how do they cope with taunting and bullying of the child?

If the child is suspected of suffering petit mal attacks he should be carefully observed at school. Petit mal may start at 5–9 years. It is uncommon and may be missed as a cause of learning difficulties. Flicking of the eyes may occur. EEG characteristically shows spike and wave 3 Hz.

The school doctor needs to know the policy on the child's ability to play football, cricket, swimming, horse riding, boxing, cycling and other activities.

If, on the other hand *the child is not coping well*, the doctor must consider other factors:

Is the child misplaced in an ordinary school because of low IQ? (one in four epileptic children are educationally subnormal).

Has the child visuospatial learning difficulties? These are the most frequent learning problems associated with epilepsy. With IQ tests it is important to include both non-verbal and verbal tests, otherwise if only verbal competence is tested, an inaccurate over-high result may be obtained.

79

What drugs is the child having? Phenobarbitone, phenytoin and sultiame all affect learning processes. Regular blood levels of anti-convulsant drugs should be estimated to check on correct dosage.

In very refractory cases admission to a *special epilepsy colony* may be recommended. Parents are often very resistant to this idea and the general practitioner can help the child by counselling the parents to accept this advice since most such institutions achieve very good results and the majority of the children are able to return home and attend ordinary schools.

Other handicaps (see also pp. 87–100)

It is often assumed that the majority of handicapped schoolchildren are receiving their education in 'special' schools, and that the staff attending such schools are especially trained for the task. However, in one South London Health Authority in 1984 there were almost 1000 (984) children of school age on the handicap register. It was somewhat surprising to find that approximately 60% were in 'special' schools whilst the remaining 40% attended normal schools. This is a welcome trend but it means that 40% of handicapped children may not be receiving appropriate specialized medical and nursing help and support.

The number of handicapped pupils in 'special' schools in 1983 were:

England	140 189
Wales	19 492
Scotland	10 871
N. Ireland	4 287

This represented 2.3% of all school children.

References

1. Davie, R., Butler, N. and Gildstein, H. (1972). *From Birth to Seven. National Child Development Study.* (London: Longmans/National Children's Bureau)
2. Reynolds, D. (1977). The delinquent school. In Hammersley, H. and Woods, P. (eds.) *The Process of Schooling.* (London: Routledge and Kegan Paul)
3. Rutter, M., Maugham, B., Mortimore, P. and Ouston, J. (1979). *15,000 Hours – Secondary Schools and Their Effects on Children.* (London: Open Book)
4. Fry, J. (1985). *Common Diseases.* (Lancaster: MTP Press)
5. Holdsworth, L. and Whitmore, K. (1974). A study of children with epilepsy attending ordinary schools. *Dev. Med. Child Neurol.,* **16,** 746
6. NCH (1984). *Children Today. A Fact File about Children in Great Britain and Northern Ireland.* (The National Children's Home: 85 Highbury Park, London, N5 1UD)

11

Learning problems

The Warnock Committee[1] estimated that up to one in five children at some time during their school lives will need some form of special educational provision. The Education Act of 1981 (implemented in 1983) aims to help the needs of these children. Each child is individually assessed and provision for his/her needs sought. This contrasts with the previous method in which the child was first categorized and then placed in an educational unit which dealt with that category of handicap. However, no extra resources have been provided. It is difficult, also, to provide a child's educational needs when the Act fails to define exactly what are the 'special educational needs'.

PROBLEMS OF LEARNING

Learning problems are very prevalent. Backwardness in reading (i.e. 2 years or more behind the chronological age) occurs in 10% of primary school children. In some inner cities this rises to 20–30%. Boys are more affected than girls.

Until recently, learning problems were not thought to be medical issues, but there is a growing need for them to be specifically diagnosed before treatment, since different conditions need different treatments. Moreover, even if the problem is a 'pure' learning problem, a case can be made out for the child to receive individual help for his particular problem rather than putting all children with differing learning problems into a general 'remedial' class.

The causes of learning problems are legion, *mental retardation* being the most common. In investigating these children the IQ must be measured.

IQ tests must be chosen which measure both verbal and non-verbal reasoning, because differences in scores between the two may have diagnostic significance. IQ tests must be chosen which do not rely upon the written word because these will penalize the score if the child cannot interpret words and letters.

Severely mentally retarded children have a lower score in the non-verbal part compared with the verbal, since the acquisition of language is more affected by environment than non-verbal skills.

Expressive language delay represents the neurodevelopmental immaturity which often spills over into delayed reading, spelling and writing skills – therefore it is important to test the *child's language*, both in expression and comprehension. If this is poor, it is expected that the verbal part of his IQ may be lower than the non-verbal part. If the child is, however, of normal intelligence, his non-verbal score should be average.

MENTAL RETARDATION

If language is delayed because of mental retardation, the non-verbal score on the IQ will also be low.

MINIMAL CEREBRAL DYSFUNCTION

10–15% of delayed learners suffer from minimal cerebral dysfunction, i.e. they are more clumsy, less co-ordinated and have visuospatial problems compared with their peers and have a cluster of 'soft' neurological signs. These children may be fair readers but atrocious spellers and their handwriting is painfully slow and illegible. (Perinatal risk factors such as apnoea are more frequent in this group.)

SENSORY LOSS

Children suffering from sensory losses also suffer from learning problems. *Partially sighted children* of normal intelligence frequently have problems of visual perception making spelling and mathematics difficult to learn (Figure 11.1). *Deaf children* are well known to have poor language, reading and spelling skills (Figure 11.2). In a European study of deaf children over 50% were unable to read and almost all had some kind of learning problem[2].

The problem of partial and intermittent hearing loss due to *glue ears* is currently the source of much controversy, particularly with regard to whether it causes learning and language delays. There is no

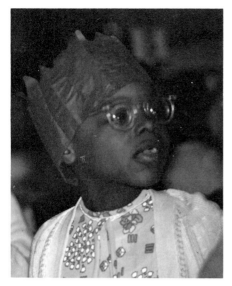

Figure 11.1   Wearing glasses . . .

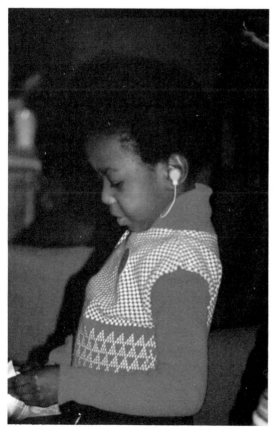

Figure 11.2   . . . and hearing aid.

doubt, many children presenting at school with poor language development will be found to be suffering a mild hearing loss from bilateral glue ears, but slow learners do not appear to have a higher prevalence of glue ears. More research is needed before this can definitely be equated with learning problems.

SOCIOEMOTIONAL DEPRIVATION

Children suffering from *conduct disorders* or from social and emotional deprivation may all present with learning problems. These learning difficulties tend to be secondary to their life patterns which are characterized by a general lack of discipline. Learning phonetic and visual perceptive skills for reading requires both a cognitive and physical discipline which they have never been taught. They fall behind their peers and, combined with a lack of encouragement and interest in their school performance by their parents, this produces a lack of motivation to the whole school process.

SPECIFIC LEARNING PROBLEM (DYSLEXIA)

When all the above causes of learning problems have been excluded there will still be a core of children who have delayed reading and spelling (Rutter[3], in the Isle of Wight, found this to be 2-7%).

This can variously be described as *dyslexia* or specific reading difficulty. *'Specific learning problem'* is the current favourite since spelling is always affected as well as reading, and it is spelling that proves more intractable to improvement than reading. Boys are more affected than girls. There is a strong family history of the same problem, usually in one or both parents. The adults are usually left with no or mild reading problem but a definite lifelong spelling deficit.

These children are usually described as having normal IQs, receiving adequate educational experience, living in a loving and stimulating home and having no sensory loss or physical handicap, yet they are 2 years or more behind their chronological age in reading and spelling. Accurate testing reveals an absence of 'soft' neurological signs.

However, tests on these children with the Pollak Tapper[4] show that the majority have either poor visual or poor auditory perceptions and memory, rarely both. These are children, par excellence, who require individual help with their own problems. Obviously 'look and say' methods of reading are unhelpful for a child with visual perception

84

problems, whilst phonetic methods will be difficult for a child with poor auditory perceptual skills.

MIXED PROBLEMS

In addition to specific conditions there are mixed problems with minimal cerebral dysfunction and social deprivation and language delay interwoven together.

References

1. Warnock, H. M. (1978). *Special Educational Needs. Report of Committee of Enquiry into the Education of Handicapped Children and Young People, 1978.* (HMSO)
2. Martin, J. A. M. and Moore, W. J. (1979). *Childhood Deafness in the European Community.* (Luxembourg: Commission of the European Community)
3. Rutter, M., Tizard, J. and Whitmore, K. (1970). *Education, Health and Behaviour.* (London: Longmans)
4. Pollak, M. and Tuchler, H. (1982). The Pollak Tapper. *Headteachers' Review,* summer

12

Handicapped children

The prevalence of handicap in the child population is difficult to quantify because the definition of handicap varies and many children have several handicaps. Thus, one half of severely mentally handicapped children have additional physical handicaps.

The National Child Development study estimated that 13% of 7-year-olds were in, or would have benefited from, special educational help[1].

Bradshaw estimated approximately 0.8% of children have a very severe mental and/or physical handicap[2]. For every *severe* handicap there will be 3-4 *moderately* handicapped children, i.e. 3% of the population.

In any cohort of handicapped children about two thirds will suffer from *mental handicap* (Figure 12.1).

Handicapped children – numbers in a practice population of 10 000 with 1000 children under 10

	Ref.	Per 1000 children under 10
Severe mental retardation (IQ below 50)	3	2.5
Moderate mental retardation (IQ 50–75)	4	30
Blind (registered)	5	0.2
Deaf (needing hearing aids)	6	2
Appreciable speech impairment (at 7 years)	7	110
Epilepsy (at 10–11 years)	6	8.4
Cerebral palsy (live births)	8	2

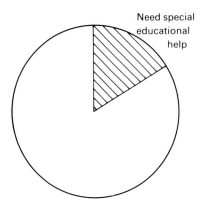

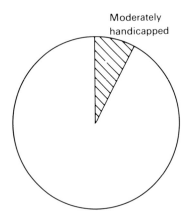

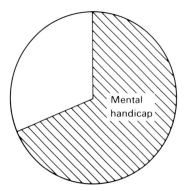

Figure 12.1   All handicapped children.

Although not strictly 'handicaps' there are many persisting and chronic disorders affecting children and the numbers of such chronic disorders per 1000 children are shown in the table.

	Per 1000 children under 10
Asthma	50
Eczema	100
Enuresis	
at 5	200
at 10	60
Squint (under supervision)	30
Headaches	120
Abdominal pains	60

There is wide difference between children in how much their handicap disables them; for example, asthma has a prevalence of 5% yet few children are appreciably handicapped. The principles of care that apply to mental handicap apply equally to physical handicaps.

BASIC NEEDS

Although they have *special* needs, handicapped children also have the *same needs* as ordinary children. A Down's syndrome baby needs Christmas just like other children (Figure 12.2).

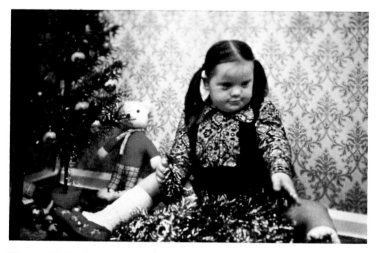

Figure 12.2 Down's syndrome at Christmas (by kind permission of *World Medicine*).

They need to be *loved and cherished*. (The painting by Velasquez in Figure 12.3 shows the dwarf, a handicapped person, honoured and cared for in the court of the little Princess.) They need to be treated as *real people* in their own right, playing a role in society, although

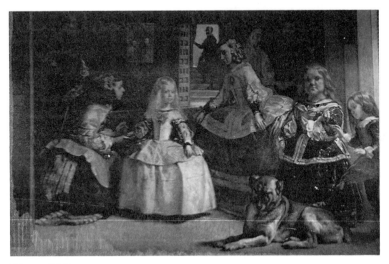

Figure 12.3

handicapped. (Figure 12.4 shows a microcephalic boy, playing the bagpipes at a strawberry fair in Brittany. The others in the band are normal.)

They need to play and *learn through play*, particularly because their mobility may be limited or a sensory system inadequate. Many public libraries have advisers in toys and play stimulation.

The boy in Figure 12.5, who has cerebral palsy, is placed on a wedge to help his head control and strengthen the tone in the upper limbs, thus enabling him to reach out and play with his toys.

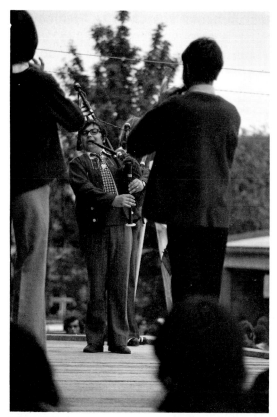

Figure 12.4

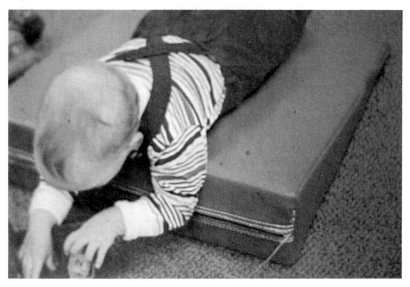

Figure 12.5   Support for head on wedge.

Tony, a mongol aged 23, has a mental age of 8–9 y. His mother realizes this and has given him a colouring book suitable for his mental age (Figure 12.6). The result is that he will sit quietly colouring this for some time, instead of restless, inconsequential behaviour if he is given material suitable for a 23-year-old.

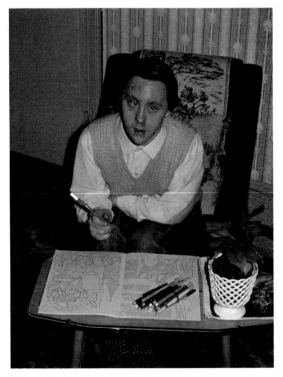

Figure 12.6

RISK FACTORS

Handicapped children are more likely to be 'at risk' than ordinary children:

more difficult to fulfil their *potential*

Cheryl has a spastic diplegia with a motor handicap but she is of normal intelligence (Figure 12.7). It proved very difficult to get acceptance to attendance at normal school. Eventually succeeded and she is doing well.

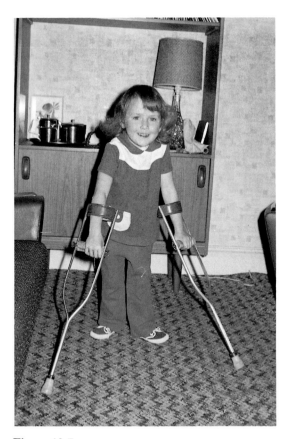

Figure 12.7

more likely to have *behaviour problems*

more likely to be *over-protected*

Anita suffered from fragile bones (fragilitas ossium) (Figure 12.8). She also suffered from a mild general delay. It was discovered that her mother kept her in a cot all day and only took her out in a pram. She was not allowed to play with her boisterous older brother – all for fear of fractures and injuries, of which she had had several. It was difficult to persuade her mother to give her normal play activities.

---

more likely to go into *care* or *residential homes*

more likely to suffer *cot deaths*

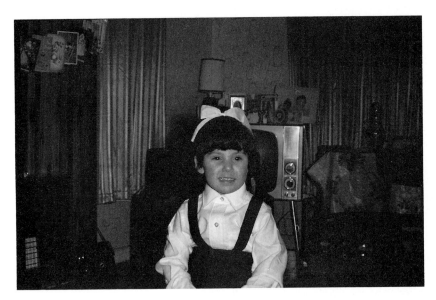

Figure 12.8

more likely to be *battered*

The *families of handicapped children* are more likely to be *'at risk'* families. Gray has shown[9] that these families are:

more likely to suffer from *marital discord*

more likely to require *psychiatric help*

more likely to *change doctors* (and get second opinions)

less likely to limit their *family size*

more likely to *move house*

HOW CAN THE FAMILY DOCTOR HELP?

He can be aware of the special risks which these children and their families run. He can be aware of the variations in attitudes and behaviour in different homes and different social classes. He can do this by continuing to see the child and family, especially at his Baby Clinic, even though they also attend the hospital or Assessment Centre.

He can encourage progress, e.g. Mongols do eventually walk. He can look for second handicaps. Squint is a common accompaniment of congenital hemiplegia (Figures 12.9 and 12.10).

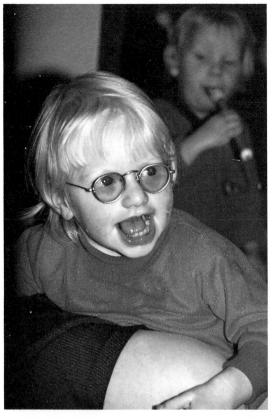

Figure 12.9 Hemiplegia and squint.

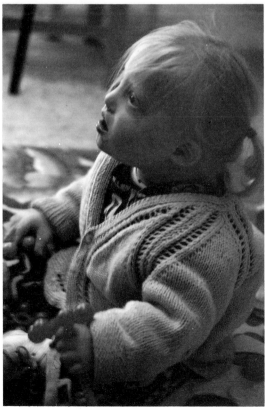

Figure 12.10 Mental
retardation and deafness.

Counselling the parents

This is delicate and strenuous work, but very worthwhile since the parents are most likely to accept support from a familiar and constant figure, i.e. the GP. There are four critical periods in the life of a handicapped child.

When the news is first told

The GP can back up what has already been mentioned. It is important to allow the parents to ask questions which are likely to include – will he walk, talk, go to school, become independent (although the baby may be only 10 days old).

After genetic counselling

One of the parents is extremely likely to feel very guilty or apportion blame. This needs talking through and marital discord will often be uncovered in this interview.

Acceptance of a 'special' school

Children attending special schools are entitled to transport to school. It is obvious to neighbours that this child is not going to the same school as most other children in the road. Many parents find this acutely embarrassing. The only real remedy is counselling work with the parents from day one, working all the time towards acceptance of the special school long before school age is reached. There are positive sides to special schools for handicapped children and the new Education Act is unlikely to alter the position for severely mentally handicapped children; they will continue to attend special schools.

When school ends

The last crisis for handicapped children and their parents is the worst. What will happen when school ends? On the whole, the facilities and support available for babies and small children with handicaps are fairly adequate, but those for adolescent and school leavers are poor. For example, in a large survey, one half of 'special' schools had no careers teachers and two thirds of the handicapped school leavers in 1980 either had no careers teachers at school or had not discussed their future with one[10]. Both the handicapped child and his parents are prone to depression at this time.

Counselling the whole family

This is a role exclusive to the family doctor and the primary team. He can notice if there is marital stress, family quarrels or if the siblings are being neglected. He can get the local Social Services to arrange some holidays and weekends away from the handicapped child. He may need to play a role in persuading the family to accept these very necessary breaks. The use of the Portage method of home stimulation can, in well chosen families, be extremely helpful, since it gives the mother (or other members of the family) a practical task. The child will achieve this task in due course and this achievement reinforces motivation to carry out the next task.

Portage is a system of home intervention based on developmental milestones. Parents are instructed to carry out a weekly programme of help and report progress. Portage was originally used for handicapped children but has been successfully used in nurseries and with 'deprived' children.

Accepting anger

The family doctor should be prepared to accept some of the anger which is part of the bereavement syndrome suffered by many parents who mourn the perfect child they expected but have not got. Not infrequently the anger is directed towards those who are 'caring' for the child, including doctors. Did he do something wrong during the labour? Was it because he gave gas and air? If the doctor had not given me iron tablets during pregnancy, would the baby have been all right? The questions may seem illogical but should be given time to be aired and answers given.

Providing all possible help

Although the general practitioner may not be the leader of the orchestra, the primary care team can ensure that Social Services and voluntary organizations are providing all the help and assistance which is available and which the parents wish to accept.

Accepting the child

The acceptance of a handicapped child is never a quick response, indeed it often takes years and sometimes is never properly accepted.

ILLUSTRATIVE CASE

Robert is a mutant trisomy-21 (Figure 12.11). Even his conception was fraught with problems. His mother, a pretty Irish Catholic girl, was aged 19 when she became engaged to John, also an Irish Catholic. The engagement was stormy, John having a tendency to stay too late in the pubs. Just when the engagement seemed likely to be broken off, Jean fell pregnant. The wedding night was marred by a quarrel brought on by the groom's drunkenness and the bride's frigidity.

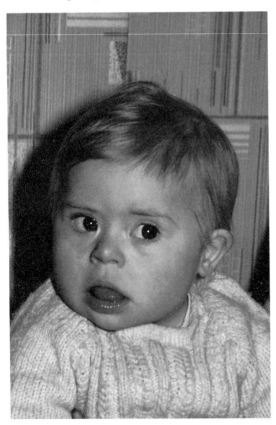

Figure 12.11

When Robert was born, after a forceps delivery which Jean described as 'agony', Down's syndrome was soon diagnosed. John went out and got 'sloshed'. Jean didn't want to bring Robert home. Eventually, some sort of family life was established. Visits by the health visitor were not accepted. Robert was not brought to the weekly clinic at the practice. Eventually, Robert needed a home visit for a chest infection. During this visit, the family doctor established that Robert had a heart lesion, was small for length, and established a relationship with the mother (over several visits) strong enough to get attendance at the baby clinic. Although Jean always came late to the clinic, to make sure that none of the other mothers would see Robert, she came.

The health visitor reported seeing Jean out shopping without Robert. She feared he might be left alone at home. This proved to be true.

John was caught for drunken driving. Counselling for his alcoholism was attempted but was unsuccessful. It was disclosed that he never took Robert out and blamed his wife for Robert.

When Robert was 3 years old the cardiologist recommended surgery. Robert died under the anaesthetic. The marriage ended in separation shortly after Robert's death. Jean returned home to Ireland and John moved away. This liaison, which was insecure from the start, was made totally unstable by the presence of a handicapped child. Neither parent ever came to terms with the handicap or with Robert as a person. Each behaved in a pattern suggested by their earlier personality types.

References

1. Pringle, M. L. K., Butler, N. R. and Davie, R. (1966). *The National Child Development Study: 11,000 7 year olds.* (London: Longman)
2. Bradshaw, J. (1975). Research and the family fund. *Concern*, **16,** 20
3. Abramowicz, H. R. and Richardson, S. A. (1975). Epidemiology of severe mental retardation in children: community studies. *Am. J. Ment. Def.*, **80,** 18
4. Kirman, B. H. (1972). *The Mentally Handicapped Child.* (London: Nelson)
5. Drillien, C. H. and Drummer, M. B. (1977). *Neurodevelopmental Problems in Early Childhood.* (Oxford: Blackwell)
6. Rutter, M., Tizard, J. and Whitmore, K. (1970). *Education, Health and Behaviour.* (London: Longman)
7. Butler, N. R., Peckham, C. and Sheridan, M. (1973). Speech defects in children aged 7, a national study. *Br. Med. J.*, **1,** 253
8. Mair, A. (1961). In Henderson, J. L. (ed.) *Cerebral Palsy in Childhood and Adolescence.* (Edinburgh: Churchill Livingstone)

9. Gray, D. P. (1977). The clinical care of handicapped children. In Hart, C. (ed.) *Child Care in General Practice*. (London: Churchill Livingstone)
10. National Children's Bureau Information Service (1980). *Highlight 44*. (Adam House, 1 Fitzroy Square, London, W1)

SECTION III

Common Clinical Problems

INTRODUCTION

There are many textbooks that cover the whole range of diseases of children. Here we aim to deal with some practical aspects of the more common clinical conditions that may cause problems in general practice.

Their management becomes easier when their nature, causes, course and outcome are known and applied. Of particular importance is the natural outcome of the condition when untreated with any specific drugs such as antibiotics.

Therefore, under each condition we aim to ask questions and provide answers.

What is the condition?

nature
frequency
causes

What is the natural history?

course and outcome
complications

What is its importance?

unpleasant symptoms
possible permanent damage

What to do?

explanation and information to parent
relief of symptoms
specific curative treatment

13

Catarrhal children

WHAT IS IT?

Nature

Almost all young children are affected by this common and well nigh inevitable syndrome (Figure 13.1). The *clinical types* do not mirror the likely *causes* (see p. 106). This leads to confusion of nomenclature and uncertainties in management. The distinct clinical types are:

coughs, colds and catarrh
croup
acute sore throats
acute chest infections
earache

Coughs, colds and catarrh

These are recurring infections of the upper respiratory tract with nasal discharge, obstruction and cough and with variable degrees of systemic upset.

Croup

Croup is a distinct infection of the larynx and adjacent tissues leading to a croaky barking cough and a variable amount of respiratory distress.

Acute sore throat

The symptoms are referrable to the throat when the child is able to complain and the appearances are of general uniform swelling and redness of tonsils and pharynx (pharyngitis) or more distinct swelling

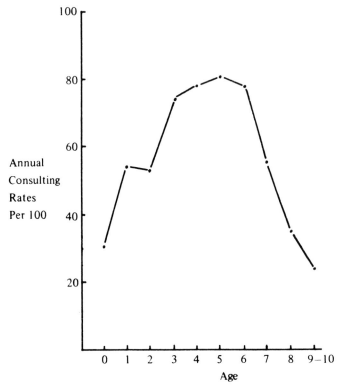

Annual
Consulting
Rates
Per 100

Age

Figure 13.1 Catarrhal children – annual consulting rates (from reference 1).

of tonsils with exudate (tonsillitis) Such distinctions are rather academic because they do not relate to specific causes.

Acute chest infections

The clinical types are *acute wheezy chests* (AWC) with generalized wheezes and cough and again varying amounts of general malaise. The child may be unaffected in spite of the wheeze or may be seriously ill with breathlessness, fever and collapse.

The other clinical type presents with irritating cough and with an area of localized moist sounds (rales and crackles) at one, or both, lung bases. This may be a localized *pneumonitis*, *pneumonia* or *bronchiolitis*.

Earache

Earache (acute otitis media) is severe enough to cause pain and distress; red drum; deafness either as significant initial symptom or persistent after acute phase is past; and occasional discharge (in 10% of attacks).

Frequency

It is likely that few children under 10 escape with less than 2 or 3 respiratory infections each year. Not all lead to consultations with the

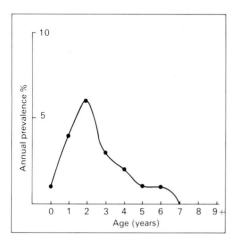

Figure 13.2   Croup – annual prevalence.

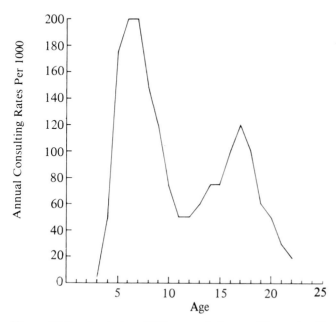

Figure 13.3   Acute tonsillitis – annual consulting rates (from reference 1).

doctor. The consulting rates depend more on mother's ability to cope than on prevalence of the infections.

There is a characteristic general pattern of prevalence for the *catarrhal child syndrome* with an appreciable prevalence in infancy, with a peak at the 4–7 year period, followed by natural decline after 8 years. *Croup* occurs almost entirely between 6 months and 3 years (Figure 13.2). *Acute throat infections* have a peak at 4–8 years and a second peak in the teens (Figure 13.3).

Causes

It is difficult to correlate distinct clinical types with definable causes. Coughs, colds, earaches, sore throats or wheezy chests may be caused by a single or a variety of pathogens or a single pathogen may cause all or some of these clinical presentations. What is evident is that even with intensive attempts at isolating causal pathogens, in no more than one third to one half will such isolation be successful. This is not important in practice as management depends more on the degrees of illness and likely natural history than on attempts to isolate bacteria or viruses.

Inability to isolate pathogens may be a fault in techniques or it may be that the conditions are not caused by infections. It may be that they represent immunological reactions to non-infective stimuli or irritants in immature respiratory tracts resulting in swelling of lymphoid tissues and mucous membranes.

Common pathogens isolated in acute respiratory infections in children

Virus
Rhinoviruses
Parainfluenzae A and B
Influenza A and B
Adenovirus
Coxsackie A and B
Respiratory syncytial virus
Herpes simplex virus

Bacteria
Streptococcus pyogenes
Streptococcus pneumoniae
Haemophilus influenzae

Even with intensive investigations pathogens are isolated in only one third of episodes.

Clinical conditions – common causal pathogens

Colds and *coughs* (pathogens isolated in less than 10% episodes)
  Rhinoviruses
  Parainfluenzae

Croup (pathogens isolated in 33% episodes)
  Parainfluenzae
  Respiratory syncytial virus

Acute throat infections (pathogens isolated in 33% episodes)
  Streptococcus pyogenes
  Parainfluenzae
  Adenovirus

Acute otitis media (pathogens isolated in less than 50% episodes)
  Streptococcus pneumoniae
  Haemophilus influenzae

Acute chest infections (pathogens isolated in about 20% episodes)
  Respiratory syncytial virus (in bronchiolitis)
  Influenza
  Parainfluenza
  Streptococcus pneumoniae

NATURAL HISTORY

Whatever the causes the natural course of these disorders is to remit and become less frequent after the age of 7–8 when colds and coughs become less frequent, tonsils shrink in size, cervical glands become impalpable and wheezy attacks infrequent[1].

Complications may occur during the periods of activity and have to be anticipated, prevented and treated whenever possible.

Acute throat infections

These rarely lead to quinsy and acute epiglottitis is very rare. A few children (5–10%) may continue to suffer recurring attacks after the age of 8 and in some there may be fresh recurring attacks in the teens, with poor general health.

Acute chest infections

These are much less severe than in the 1930s and 1940s and permanent damage with chronic suppurative lung infections is almost unknown, except in cystic fibrosis or in children with immunological disorders.

'Asthma'

Asthma with persistent recurring attacks of wheezing occurs only in 5–10% of childhood wheezers. However, there are a small number of children who do suffer severe bouts of airways obstruction and many of these will continue to have attacks, but many of these will cease having attacks by the time they reach their teens.

Natural history of chest wheezing in children

Incidence – 20–25% children suffer one or more attacks of wheezing[1]

1–2 attacks only	60%
Wheezing at 10–15 years	10%
Wheezing as adults	5%

The spectrum of severity and significance of chest wheezing is great. At one end is the child with only one or two wheezy attacks with respiratory infections and no further troubles. At the other end of the spectrum are children with frequent or constant wheezing and severe distress and disability – these are infrequent. In between there are children with wheezy chests over a period of some years, from 4 to 10 years of age, with eventual natural cessation. Should all 'wheezers' be labelled as 'asthmatics'? They can if parents are reassured of good natural outcome but it may be best to call them wheezy attacks in hypersensitive chests.

Earache (*acute otitis media*)

The natural history is reassuring. Following the peak at 4–8 years, attacks then cease (Figure 13.4). Even in children with recurring attacks of otitis media permanent hearing loss is unusual[1].

The *inflamed eardrum* may take up to 6 weeks to return to normal and there will be some hearing loss at this time. *Persistent ear discharge*, now rare, in less than 5% of attacks, can lead to scarring of the the drum but even this does not necessarily lead to appreciable hearing loss. Persistent collections of thick mucus (*glue ear*) do cause deafness whilst they are present but even these tend to resolve given time – but how much time should be allowed if there is deafness that interferes with development and learning?

Glue ear is not a new syndrome. It was termed 'catarrhal otitis media' in the past and was left to resolve naturally or treated by myringotomy and adenoidectomy.

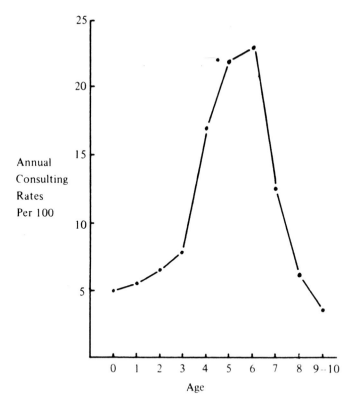

Figure 13.4 Acute otitis media – annual consulting rates (from reference 1).

It is important to *test hearing* approximately 6 weeks after an acute otitis media and to follow up children if hearing is not normal. In this way those with persistent deafness will be discovered and treated.

SIGNIFICANCE AND IMPORTANCE

The various components of the catarrhal child syndrome are of very considerable importance in general practice, because:

they are so prevalent
they cause unpleasant symptoms and ill health
they may lead to permanent functional damage

Effective management has to be a combination of sound clinical common sense and judgement, steering a course between giving nature a chance and using modern medical drugs and surgical technologies.

WHAT TO DO?

Good management involves care of the parents as well as the child, therefore it must include:

explanation and support of the parents
relief of symptoms
specific treatments as and when indicated

Explanation and support of the parents

Recurring and persisting respiratory infections with poor health are matters of concern to parents. They naturally become anxious. Their anxieties are increased by grandparents, teachers and friends who imply that 'something must be done!'

It is important to explain to parents the nature of the condition and its likely course, with recurring attacks over a few years with eventual cessation and with no permanent ill-effects. Management of attacks becomes easier if parents understand, are reassured and become confident in treating each attack themselves.

Relief of symptoms

There is much that can be done to relieve the common symptoms of cough, nasal obstruction, sore throats, earaches and chest wheezing.

coughs can be relieved by warm drinks and some simple linctus

croup by steam inhalations

earache and sore throats by analgesics

chest wheezing by antispasmodics.

Specific treatments

These are use of antibiotics, tonsillectomy and/or adenoidectomy and insertion of ear grommets.

Antibiotics

These should be used with discretion and for definite indications. They should not be used automatically and without consideration for all sore throats, all earaches and all wheezy chests. Many are unlikely to be caused by antibiotic-sensitive pathogens and many attacks will resolve without antibiotics.

Unless there are good reasons for using them such as:

severe infection with considerable systemic disturbance

severe local symptoms

previous history of problems and complications

family history of serious ear disease or chronic chest disease

then it is justifiable to delay for 1–3 days to see if the condition begins to improve naturally. Non-use of antibiotics makes it important, as in use of antibiotics, to follow-up the children until the ears, throat and chest return to normal.

Tonsillectomy and/or adenoidectomy

Recurring attacks of acute otitis media with persistent deafness and glue ear are indications to consider adenoidectomy. Repeated attacks of true tonsillitis if persisting after age of 8 make tonsillectomy a possibility.

Insertion of grommets

This is left to the ENT surgeon, but one cannot help wondering whether they are all really necessary and whether the results justify their insertion. The present debate as to when or if to use grommets continues. It is sensible to avoid a procedure with some risks, albeit few, unless there is appreciable persistent or intermittent hearing loss with poor speech development or failure at school. In selected cases there are good results but in many the procedure yields uncertain results.

Reference

1. Fry, J. (1985). *Common Diseases*. (Lancaster: MTP Press)

14

Tummy aches

WHAT IS IT?

Nature

'Tummy ache' in a child is a non-specific symptom that covers a wide spectrum of possible causes. It is never insignificant and never 'imaginary'. It is a child's unformed message that all is not well, inside or outside the abdomen.

The spectrum of possible causes is wide ranging from emotional and behavioural problems to acute life-threatening catastrophes. Classification is crude into non-organic and organic groups.

Non-organic

Stress reactions to home, school and other factors may be creating turmoil and upsets within the child's psyche. *Associated features* may be sleep problems, not eating, bowel disturbances, stealing and general 'misbehaviour' (see also pages 39–48).

'Periodic syndrome' refers to bouts of abdominal pain often with vomiting and headache (in older children). It is suggested that it may be a forerunner of migraine in later life, but most cease to have attacks with no further problems.

Food allergy is currently a popular explanation of tummy ache of undetermined cause. It may be, but in practice it is difficult to define the causal culprit and to withdraw it from the diet. Nevertheless, it should be considered and foods such as cow's milk, chocolates, nuts, cheese and artificial ingredients of modern foods might be suspected.

Organic

Intra-abdominal causes, if present, are generally serious and of immediate concern, such as:

acute gastroenteritis
acute appendicitis
strangulated hernia
intestinal obstruction from various causes
strangulated hernia and torsion of testis in older boys
intussusception in infants
urinary tract infections
sickle cell crisis

In *extra-abdominal* conditions tummy ache is a common presentation. Acute otitis media and more diffuse respiratory infections may present as tummy ache as can any general condition in its early stages including measles and other specific fevers in their prodromal stages.

Frequency

Tummy ache can only present if the child is able to complain of it. Screaming infants often are believed by their parents to be suffering from 'wind' or 'colic', or constipation. So they may, but who can be sure?

The prevalence of abdominal pain in children has its peak between 3 and 8 years but it continues at a lower but significant level thereafter, sometimes into adulthood in some individuals.

Tummy ache in young children is equally prevalent in boys and girls. Abdominal pains are much more frequent in girls between 10 and 15 years, presumably related to the onset of menstruation and its associated problems (Figure 14.1).

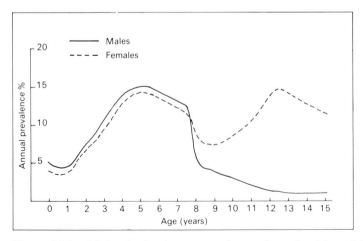

Figure 14.1 Abdominal pains – annual prevalence in girls and boys.

NATURAL HISTORY

The occasional bout of tummy ache is more likely to be caused by a specific organic condition that resolves with the causal condition.

Recurrent bouts of tummy ache in young children are more likely to be non-organic – although in girls at menarche and after they are probably related to their monthly cycles.

The non-organic tummy aches of children at 3–8 years of age tend to disappear and do not return.

Only a proportion will grow up and suffer from migraine, irritable bowel syndromes and psychosomatic disorders, probably less than 10–15%.

SIGNIFICANCE AND IMPORTANCE

Tummy ache is a cause of anxiety to parents and doctors. Parents are unsure of the nature and significance of recurring bouts and are concerned that the sudden unexpected attack may be due to 'appendicitis'. So it may be and it must never be neglected by the doctor. The 'missed appendix' can have disastrous consequences and it is missed usually because of failure to suspect it and failure to see and examine, and possibly re-examine, the child with recent abdominal pain.

Beware of the quiet, still and ill child who complains of abdominal pain and who has vomited – even if the abdominal signs may be indefinite and undramatic.

WHAT TO DO?

Think – in every child with abdominal pains the doctor must consider the possible diagnoses based on the presenting situation and from his past knowledge of the child and family.

Listen – give the mother the chance to tell the story; the answer usually reveals itself from the history.

Assess – now the possibilities must be carefully considered:

    is it a new or recurring condition?
    is the child ill?
    does there appear to be an intra-abdominal condition?
    is there any likely extra-abdominal cause?
    are there any investigations required – now or later?

Act –

is immediate hospital admission necessary?

if not, how to manage the acute case?

apart from antibiotics for specific condition such as respiratory or urinary tract infections there are few indications for medication.

give mother clear instructions and explanation on what it is, what is likely to happen and what to look for and report if course is not as predicted.

arrange for follow-up or for some continuing contract.

in the recurring and non-acute case consider:

personal and family situations
long-term management and advice
need for further investigations
referral to consultant – this may be to seek special expertise and experience or to reassure the mother.

15

Bowel problems – too much or too little

WHAT IS IT?

There is a great spectrum of normality of frequency and consistency of bowel action (Figure 15.1). It may be normal for a breast-fed baby to have bowels open after every feed or only once or twice a week. It may be normal for infants and older children likewise to have their bowels open at varying frequencies. Providing that the child is well the frequency or infrequency of bowel movements are unimportant.

It is of interest to note that the diagnosis of 'constipation' is most prevalent in the young and in the old (Figure 15.2). There are many possible causes of 'diarrhoea' and 'constipation'. A list of the more common ones serves only as an *aide-mémoire*.

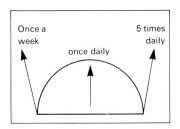

Figure 15.1   Frequency of bowel actions.

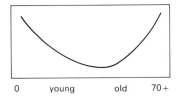

Figure 15.2   Prevalence of constipation.

Diarrhoea

physiological

acute gastroenteritis

intolerances to lactose, cow's milk and other food ingredients (these often follow attack of gastroenteritis)

117

frequent hard green stools in underfed infant

spurious due to fecal impaction

note: uncommon specific infections, such as salmonella, campylo-bacter, *giardia lamblia*, and worms especially in immigrants and travellers from overseas

note: diarrhoea as early feature in the acute surgical abdomen, i.e. appendicitis and intussusception

Very rare are:
  coeliac disease (note wasting of gluteal muscles and consistency
    of stools – chalky/fatty)
  fibrocystic disease
  ulcerative colitis
  Crohn's disease

Constipation

physiological

fecal impaction

fecal soiling and encopresis

very rare:
  Hirschsprung's disease
  threadworms

SIGNIFICANCE AND IMPORTANCE

In general practice there is a predominance of common and less ser-ious conditions over the selected clinical material in hospital practice. Nevertheless, the general practitioner has to be prepared to consider less common and more serious disorders.

Although most cases of *acute diarrhoea* (and sickness) are short, self-limiting, safe disorders endemic in all communities and at all social levels, in infants a few cases will be severe enough to cause fluid and electrolyte disturbance requiring urgent hospital care.

The more sudden and recent the change in bowel habits the more significant the situation and the more care and attention demanded from the practitioner.

Dehydration in infants

The younger the infant the more dangerous are effects of fluid loss from diarrhoea and vomiting. The best guide to assess fluid loss is loss of weight – this may be difficult to measure at home.

Useful clinical features of dehydration are:

skin – loss of turgor and mottling
fontanelle – depression
eyes – sunken
peripheral pulses – rapid and poor volume
mental state (degrees) – lethargy, prostration, coma

WHAT TO DO?

The general state of the child is much more important than the state of the bowels.

Is the child well or sick?
Is the child active or still?
Is the child crying or quiet?

The state of the parents and the home will influence management and advice. It may be safer for some infants with diarrhoea, with non-coping parents and poor home conditions, to be admitted to hospital even if apparently well.

A.B. a baby of 4 months of Nigerian parents. M.P. visited for diarrhoea and vomiting. Baby was fine but there were 14 adults in the room. Candles and incense were burning and various gods were being incited to achieve a cure. A.B. was admitted for social reasons.

Enquire about the family history of recent gastrointestinal disorders and of travel overseas.

Diarrhoea

Acute

There is no specific treatment necessary with medicines or antibiotics. Emphasis on diet will suffice in most cases. No solids for 24–48 h, but give clear fluids (with teaspoon of sugar and pinch of salt to a pint of water) even if vomiting. Do **not** give milk. For a short, sharp attack, there is no need for special electrolyte–glucose preparations. Admit if the child is dehydrated or if diarrhoea is prolonged (over 48 h).

Chronic

Persistent loose stools may be normal if present for some time and if child is well.

Recent and prolonged

Consider possible lactose or cow's milk intolerance. If it is persistent with sickly child, consider more serious conditions such as malabsorption syndromes.

Constipation

Reassure and advise on higher roughage diet if child is well and condition has been present for some time.

Acute constipation may be associated with anal fissure or be secondary to feverish condition with some dehydration.

The case may present as a screaming child and diagnosis can only be made on rectal examination, which usually produces a watery stool in gastroenteritis.

Laxatives are unhelpful – they work slowly and cause colicky abdominal pains.

With fecal impaction, glycerine suppositories will relieve the condition but patience and persistence required.

Make arrangements for follow-up and supervision on diet and home management.

16

The feverish child

WHAT IS IT?

Fever is *not* a specific disorder requiring specific treatment. Fever is a non-specific natural response to infection. It has many possible causes and in the majority of feverish children no cause is ever found, and the bout is short and self-limiting.

Who gets it?

All children may become feverish but the greatest prevalence is in infants and in early school years.

What happens?

One half of feverish children[1] are well within 24–48 h. Another 12% are well in the next 24–48 h. In feverish infants (under 2 years) 5–10% have a significant bacterial infection.

SIGNIFICANCE AND IMPORTANCE

The significance of its course relates to the cause. Febrile convulsions are of concern to parents and doctors but are uncommon, occurring in less than 1% of febrile attacks in young children. Febrile convulsions occur in children prone to convulse. Normal (non-prone) children will not convulse even with very high fever.

The height of the fever is an uncertain predictor of seriousness of the underlying cause and may be an individual reaction to non-specific infections. *But* the higher the fever the more likely it is to be a treatable bacterial infection.

WHAT TO DO?

Try and decide on the cause of fever, but note that in the great majority of cases (75%) no honest label can be attached.

Be prepared to wait for 1–2 days before making a diagnosis. Most will be resolving spontaneously or the cause may become more apparent by then.

Explain and re-explain and re-re-explain to parents that fever is not a disease but a natural normal bodily protective response that should not be discouraged. It may be helpful to explain that the fever 'burns up the bugs'.

Do *not* treat 'fever' with:

antibiotics – unless there is a good reason

aspirin or paracetamol – unless there are indications

Do advise that parents can relieve symptoms by:

removing layers of clothes

giving fluids + +

tepid sponging

Decide on a *plan of management* that includes:

definition of likely course and this should be explained to parents

continuing observation by parents

reporting of unexpected features

follow-up by seeing the child or by telephone report or by assessment by practice nurse.

Treat specific cause if known, but specific treatment with antibiotics is necessary in a minority. These may be otitis media, tonsillitis, chest infections, urinary tract infections.

The indications for antibiotics are individual for doctor and child. Some doctors will use antibiotics more liberally. In general, their indications should relate to the degree of the presenting illness and its presumed nature and cause, to past history of previous attacks or illnesses and health of child, to social and family circumstances and on opportunities for follow-up.

Be prepared to *admit to hospital* if:

no improvement within 2–3 days unless obvious reason

if child is very ill and toxic

if there is any suggestion of a major disease such as meningitis

if it is the child's first febrile convulsion or the convulsion is prolonged (over 15 min)

Reference

1. McCrutchem, M. L. (1985). The febrile infant. *J. Fam. Pract.*, **20**, 584

17

Spots and rashes

WHAT ARE THEY?

In practice there are two main groups of rashes in children

those in which a diagnostic label can be attached
those in which no diagnostic label is possible

Even when a diagnostic label is possible, the *causes* often are unclear and uncertain.

Skin disorders are prevalent at all ages but particularly so in infancy and childhood (Figure 17.1). The age–prevalence rates of common skin conditions show the high rates in childhood of most conditions (Figure 17.2).

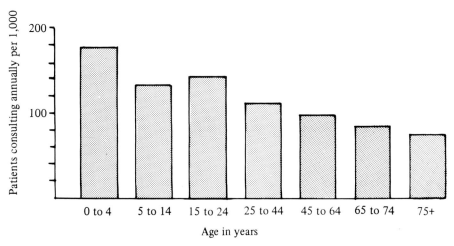

Figure 17.1 Age prevalence of skin disorders (from reference 1).

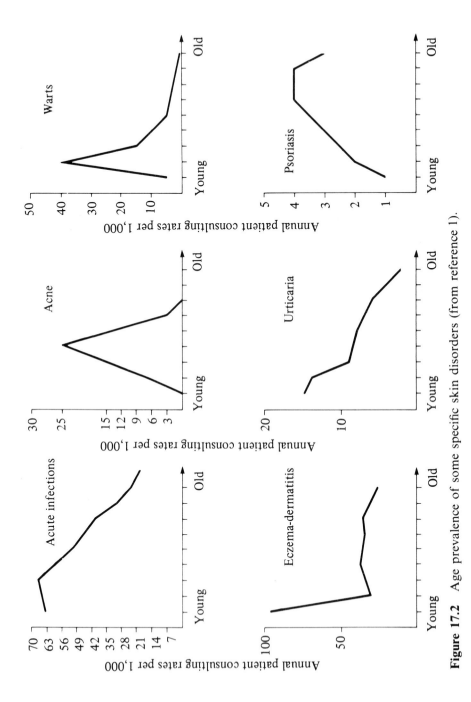

Figure 17.2 Age prevalence of some specific skin disorders (from reference 1).

126

Relative frequency of common skin conditions in children

	%		%
Infections	35	*Napkin area rashes*	10
warts		contact dermatitis	
impetigo		candidiasis	
boils, pustules, paronychia			
scabies		*Transient – unlabelled*	10
fungal		? viral	
pediculosis		? allergic	
herpetic			
Eczema – dermatitis	20	*Urticaria*	5
atopic		allergies – uncertain cause	
seborrhoeic		popular (bites)	
		drug sensitivities	
Specific fevers	10		
chicken pox		Others	10
measles		milia	
rubella		psoriasis	
roseola		pityriasis rosea	
scarlet fever		birth marks, naevi	

SIGNIFICANCE AND IMPORTANCE

Transient rashes occur in transient disorders such as infections. Persistent or recurring rashes occur in children who are individually prone or susceptible as in eczema or urticaria. Persistent rashes such as psoriasis and eczema may be difficult to control and can cause great anxiety for parents.

WHAT TO DO?

Because there are few specific 'cures' of skin disorders, their management will vary with the views of the doctor on the nature of the condition and his/her beliefs of the effectiveness of available therapeutic agents.

Since the true aetiology of most common skin conditions is uncertain, their management should be based on commonsense principles rather than at attempts at specific cures.

Although topical corticosteroids and antibiotics are the most widely used preparations, they should *never* be used over time. Older and blander ointments, creams and lotions should not be despised.

SPECIFIC CONDITIONS

Infections

Impetigo

Local antibiotics such as chlortetracycline, flucloxallin and fusidic acid are useful, *but* if the impetigo is widespread it is kinder to the child and parent to use a systemic antibiotic, such as penicillin or erythromycin, and so avoid the distress of bathing and applying creams.

Boils, paronychia

Local applications are of little value. A short course of systemic antibiotic is very effective.

Warts

Do not treat unless pressurized by parents and if so remember warts disappear in time. Start with local application of preparations of salicylic acid, then go on to cryotherapy (frozen carbon dioxide or nitrogen) and only finally consider currettage for plantar and other stubborn warts.

Scabies

This is not an easy diagnosis, is often missed and labelled 'papular urticaria' or 'eczema'. Instruct on family hygienic measures and on applications of benzyl benzoate (stings) or gamma benzene hexachloride (less stinging).

Fungal

Fungal infections are usually caught from cats and dogs. If they are localized, Whitfield's ointment (mixture of benzoic and salicylic acids) is very effective. If the infection is widespread, use oral griseofulvin for at least 1 month.

Herpetic infections

Few need any specific treatment.

Eczema – dermatitis

Seborrhoeic

This is common in infancy as cradle cap and more extensive rashes – usually well controlled by washing off scales and applying diluted corticosteroids such as hydrocortisone 0.1–0.5% or betamethosone 1 in 10.

Atopic eczema

Atopic eczema is stubborn and resistant. Onset occurs at 2–18 months but most cases improve after the age of 2 and few cases persist into adult life. Note that in a few children cases may be produced or aggravated by food allergy, notably wheat and cereals. The basic principles of management are:

avoid soap and use emulsifying ointment instead

use diluted corticosteroids as creams or ointments

do not be afraid of a short intensive course of systemic steroids for severe attacks

sedation with antihistamines is useful at night during exacerbations

Napkin rashes

There are two types of napkin rash – contact dermatitis and candidiasis.

Contact dermatitis

This is the most common type caused by contact with ammoniacal alkaline urine as the irritant.

Therefore napkins should be changed frequently and left off whenever socially possible. Barrier creams such as zinc and castor oil act as preventives, and a small amount of boric acid $\frac{1}{2}$–1% neutralizes the alkaline urine. For an acute bout corticosteroid creams are effective.

Candidiasis

This may be superimposed on a napkin dermatitis. It is redder and brighter than dermatitis and involves flexural creases. It is controlled by nystatin cream.

Urticaria

Its cause is usually unknown, and although dramatic it tends to be self-limiting. The most important part of management is to explain the diagnosis to parents and reassure that it is non-infective and will clear within days.

The benefits of antihistamines are questionable but systemic steroids may be necessary in severe attacks.

No treatment apart from reassuring explanation is required for:
milia
strawberry naevus
pityriasis rosea
alopecia areata
granuloma annulare
erythema nodosum
most warts

18

Fits and funny turns

By **Dr Peter Robson,** Senior Lecturer in Paediatric Neurology, King's College Hospital, London

'Fits and funny turns' is a convenient phrase to describe *short periods of altered behaviour (often stereotyped) of such frequency, or persistence, or of such a bizarre nature that they cause concern to the child, parents, teachers or doctors.*

Most funny turns are not epileptic (see Table 18.1): the commonest

Table 18.1 *Non-epileptic funny turns*

Temper tantrums
Breath-holding attacks
Faints and syncopies
Benign paroxysmal vertigo
Migraine
Tics
Ritualistic movements
Night terrors
Nightmares
Sleepwalking
Munchausen-by-proxy
Individual or epidemic mass hysteria

disturbance is probably the tic, occurring in some 12% to 18% of the child population at some stage in development, and most commonly affect the eyes, face and neck movements[1]. Head banging or other rhythmic motor habits were reported in up to 20% of unselected attenders at paediatric outpatients[2]. However, some funny turns, particularly breath-holding attacks, reflex bradycardia (both types developing in response to pain, fear, or being thwarted) and migraine may act as trigger mechanisms provoking epileptic seizures in susceptible children and particularly the under-5-year-olds.

Parental reactions to the first few episodes may act as behaviour modification reinforcers, thus increasing the frequency and persistence of an otherwise transient behaviour pattern, such as temper tantrums, breath-holding, tics, ritualistic movements, and sleep disturbances.

Phasic alterations in behaviour are more common in children with mental impairment, sensory handicaps (especially blindness), and communication disorders: this is partly the result of clustering of several clinical features of brain dysfunction independent of its cause, and partly the effect of slow development keeping the child longer in the 6- to 36-month developmental age range, in which behaviour regarded as abnormal later in life is normal.

Children do not always put a turn on for the doctor and therefore interrogation of the parents or others who have *witnessed* the attacks must be thorough; a useful ploy is to ask them to mime the event, once they have indicated the preceding events, time of onset, and behaviour after the attack has ceased. There may be multiple causes, and the apparent immediate trigger may be only the last of a series in which the order of the causal events changes from one attack to the next. Reliance on parental history does lead to erroneous diagnosis in some instances; some families have specific complaints to signal unhappiness such as a 'sore throat' (rapidly cured by one paracetamol tablet), phasic abdominal pain[3], or headache[4], and a child may find that an accidental behaviour pattern produced the desired parental concern and was therefore repeated: reported phasic alterations in a child's behaviour which could be interpreted as a seizure, can result in a child being treated for epilepsy (usually quite ineffectually – thus ensuring frequent hospital visits) when the real diagnosis is a family disturbance producing the Munchausen-by-proxy-syndrome[5].

A short description of an extensive subject must be incomplete and the following headings are suggested as a simple framework to record the sequence of events.

Antecedents

Unexpected pain, loss of toy, parental response to negativism – (breath-holding, temper tantrum, reflex bradycardia); pyrexia, hypoglycaemia (seizures of any sort); anxiety provokes tics or makes them more obvious; previous illness with vomiting or diarrhoea may precede attacks of vertigo, or may have been treated with anti-emetic agents such as metoclopramide which is more likely to provoke a dystonic reaction in a child than in an adult.

Onset

Gradual onset in breath-holding, temper tantrum, masturbation, and focal seizures (not always) with occasions in which attacks fail to develop fully; *sudden onset* in grand mal, reflex bradycardia, and petit mal.

Features during attack

Immediate loss of consciousness in grand mal and rapidly progressing focal fits with secondary generalization; *late loss of consciousness* in breath-holding, reflex bradycardia; *blue face* in breath-holding, and grand mal; *white face* – bradycardia, vertigo, focal fits; *red face* – breath-holding, masturbation, focal fits. *Cessation of movement without loss of muscle tone* – masturbation, true petit mal, aura of focal seizure. *Flops to floor at start of attack* – reflex bradycardia, vertigo, atypical petit mal, atonic seizure. *Falls stiffly* – grand mal, myoclonic seizure. *Eyes deviated upwards and limbs stiff* – grand mal, dystonic reaction to drugs. *Complex stereotyped purposeful movements* – tics, onset of focal fit.

Post-attack behaviour

Sleeping, drowsiness, headache, or Todd's palsy for many minutes (usually hours) indicate a generalized epilepsy. Sudden recovery of normal behaviour is seen in true behaviour problems and in true petit mal.

In nocturnal attacks, recall of the events is unusual in sleepwalking, night terrors and grand mal seizures. Recall is usually reported in nightmares and sometimes in benign focal seizures.

Time of day

Some behaviours are characteristically seen in normal children at specific times of day such as rocking and head-banging as a pre-sleep ritual. Temper tantrums may be provoked by meal-time or potty-time battles of wills. Hypoglycaemia may occur before or half to two hours after meals, and, because short-acting anticonvulsants are often given at meal-times, low blood levels may produce clustering of typical epileptic or of partially controlled attacks an hour or two before or after meals.

Recurrences

Benign paroxysmal vertigo is so named because the attacks occur in clusters of several days duration with attack-free intervals of 2 to 3 weeks in between. The paroxysms become increasingly milder with longer intervals between the paroxysms until the sequence ends after 2 to 4 cycles. Migraine-related conditions tend to have a 4- to 6-week periodicity, but this is not invariable. Some behaviour patterns seem to be time-locked into the maternal menstrual cycle. Other stress-related patterns may occur at weekends or schooldays, or just at the beginning of term. As seizures may also be stress related, this sort of periodicity does not exclude epilepsy.

Age ranges

First six to nine months; seizures due to brain hypoxia and trauma, congenital malformations and metabolic diseases; infantile spasms (salaam attacks). *First three years;* breath-holding, reflex bradycardia, temper tantrums, febrile seizures, rocking, head-banging. *Fourth to tenth years;* night terrors and nightmares. *Eleven to fourteen years;* sleepwalking.

The epilepsies can occur at any age with the familial febrile and the reflex anoxic (bradycardia) triggered attacks clustered during the first three to five years.

Management

The type of questions asked by the doctor often give the parents some idea of the benign nature of the condition, its developmental basis and its good outcome. In the absence of severe family disturbances this, or a more formal explanation, may be all that is needed. The general practitioner is in a better position to decide about disturbed family dynamics than a paediatrician, and, if the parents consent, the local family and child psychiatry department should be involved.

THE EPILEPSIES

These are defined as *an episodic disturbance of brain function charac-terized by brief, repeated, and stereotyped alterations of behaviour, often associated with impairment of consciousness.* About 5% of children suffer seizures at some time in their lives, and the majority occur in the first 5 years and have a good prognosis. *Parents are not aware of this and think their child is dying when they witness the first seizure;* this impression remains with them producing great anxiety, which needs to be considered in the management of the child and his or her family.

The adult classification of seizures into generalized and partial (focal) is not easy to apply in the very young (Table 18.2). Neonates may simply have apnoeic attacks or become rigid or atonic: because of the relative instability of the young brain, focal attacks may rapidly become generalized, and the focal origin not be recognized until an aura lasts long enough to be identified as such.

Table 18.2 *Epilepsies*

Generalized
   Motor – tonic–clonic (major, or grand mal)
       – atonic (drop attacks), tonic, myoclonic
       – infantile spasms (infantile myoclonic epilepsy)
   Absences – classical petit mal
Partial (focal)
   simple – motor, sensory, autonomic
   complex – psychomotor (temporal lobe)
   – any of these may become secondarily generalized

In the majority of children, seizures of short duration (less than 10 minutes), in the absence of developmental delay or persistent neuro-logical signs, have a good overall prognosis – some 90% ultimately becoming seizure-free by their 'teens.

The commonest form is the *febrile seizure*, occurring in some 3% to 4% of children usually during the first 4 years of life. In order not to confuse them with idiopathic epilepsy triggered by pyrexia, the defi-nition includes factors such as occurrence only during a pyrexial ill-ness, short-lived (less than 5 seconds) symmetrical tonic or clonic attack with rapid recovery, and a history of similar febrile attacks in close relatives. Repeated fits during the same febrile episode do not invalidate the febrile seizure diagnosis, but there is an increased chance of recurrence when compared with the single seizure variety. Reducing the pyrexia by cooling and paracetamol is the management of choice.

Phenobarbitone sodium is commonly used as an anticonvulsant for infants; the long half-life allows it to be given once daily in the evening, but it can exacerbate the overactivity of the toddler and produce behaviour problems. There is a trend to replace it by sodium valproate, but the medication then has to be given two or three times per day (Table 18.3).

Table 18.3 *Anticonvulsant dosages* (in mg/kg body weight per day)

Phenobarbitone	4–6	Gen. and partial.
Sodium valproate	20–35	Gen., partial and absences.
Carbamezapine	10–20	Gen. and partial.
Phenytoin	7–10	Generalized only.
Ethosuximide	20–40	Absences only.
Nitrazepam	0.5–2.0	Myoclonic and minor attacks.
Clonazepam	0.05–2.0	Myoclonic and minor attacks.

Attacks triggered by breath-holding, or reflex bradycardia are usually short clonic episodes with rapid recovery.

Neonatal seizures are the next most frequent (about 1.2%), and have origins in the biochemical and hypoxic problems of the newborn. The treatment depends on the cause and has to be instituted quickly to prevent permanent brain dysfunction.

Other forms of epilepsy are rare; true *petit mal* (0.3%) has its peak incidence at about 5 years but with a spread of from 3 to 12 years; *idiopathic grand mal* and *temporal lobe seizures* are clinically discernable from about 5 years onwards and usually appear for the first time later in childhood. *Benign focal seizures* tend to occur during the night with twitches of the face interfering with swallowing and speech with spread to one upper limb, and occasionally followed by a grand mal attack. A unilateral focal spike discharge is seen on the e.e.g. which disappears during the 'teens. *Minor epilepsy* refers to momentary loss of consciousness associated with motor phenomena – usually myoclonic jerks or atonic (drop) attacks – which differentiates it from petit mal; serious underlying brain abnormalities make it a difficult condition to treat. *Infantile spasms* (salaam attacks) are a rare but specific form of epilepsy occurring in the first year and are often confused with attacks of colic; the attacks are sudden repeated episodes of myoclonus causing the infant to flex the trunk and frequently cry out: it is a feature of structural brain abnormalities such as tuberose sclerosis (white leaf-shaped spots on skin) or encephalopathies of any origin presenting in the first 6 to 12 months of life. The investigation and management are initially hospital-based.

THE FIRST SEIZURE

The most likely cause of a first seizure in a 1 to 5-year-old will be an upper respiratory tract infection with the resultant pyrexia being the trigger; the attack will be simple (symmetrical, single and short-lived), and the child will have recovered from it by the time the doctor visits. Should it persist for more than 10 to 15 minutes, then it must be halted by rectal diazepam which works almost as quickly as intravenous injection[6]; this masks the signs of rapid recovery which is the hallmark of a true, mild febrile attack, but febrile seizures lasting more than 20 minutes are associated with later temporal lobe epilepsy, and the need to halt the attack takes priority.

The clinical skills of the family's physician are all important in the decision to send the child to hospital. Probably, when in doubt, the child should be investigated, as pyrexia and seizures are early features of meningitis and encephalitis. The decision to use antibiotics for the pyrexia needs careful consideration too; unless there is an obvious bacterial infection (many upper respiratory tract infections are viral), the antibiotic will have no definite effect and could delay the diagnosis of bacterial meningitis.

As a rule, the first mild febrile fit is not treated. The exceptions might be complex fits (long, or repeated during the same illness), doubt about the true febrile nature, and excessive parental anxiety. Neonatal seizures, and possibly all first seizures in infants, warrant hospital investigation because of the rapid deterioration in small infants and the possibility that biochemical, structural or inflammatory brain lesions are responsible. The first grand mal tends to occur after the age of 5 years; an inter-ictal e.e.g. will be normal in 40%. Good control with carbamezapine, valproate, or phenytoin is a good prognostic feature, but there is a recurrence risk of about 50% in all non-pyrexial childhood seizures, and this risk is not altered by medication[7]. Cerebral tumours are very rare, tend to be cerebellar or brain stem in this age group and epilepsy is seldom the single presenting feature even in the supratentorial lesions. It is therefore logical to assume that, in the absence of skin lesions of a neuroectodermatosis or evidence of pre-existing brain dysfunction, all first grand mal attacks are idiopathic epilepsy. Where possible, an inter-ictal e.e.g. recording not

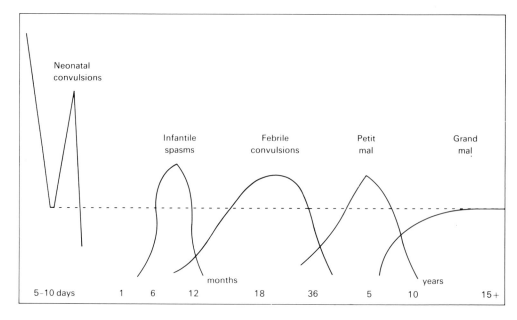

Figure 18.1 Fits – age at onset and peaks (after O'Donohoe[9]).

complicated by anticonvulsant therapy should be obtained before deciding on the appropriateness of drug therapy.

Recurrent seizures not easily controlled by anticonvulsants, and/or associated with additional facets of brain dysfunction are best dealt with in a unit specializing in paediatric neurological and neuro-developmental problems.

Status epilepticus is fortunately a very uncommon occurrence. A grand mal based status is most likely in the first five years of life. It is one occasion in which treatment precedes diagnosis: continuous seizures lasting more than 10 minutes are associated with secondary hypoxic brain dysfunction, and status lasting 30 to 60 minutes produces additional severe systemic disturbances with resultant resistance to treatment and increasing brain damage[8]. The normal principles underlying management of an unconscious patient apply – maintain oxygenation by ensuring an adequate airway and then control the seizures with diazepam (intravenously or rectally), before referral to hospital for further acute management and search for the conditions underlying the status. Status can also occur in minor motor epilepsy and in petit mal, giving a mixed and variable picture of overactivity, restlessness, drowsiness, twitches, drop attacks, tremor, phasic ataxia, which may stop spontaneously, or produce episodes of grand mal.

Single drug therapy is easier to manage and produces fewer side-effects than multiple drug therapy.

Phenobarbitone, phenytoin, nitrazepam and clonazepam have long half-lives and can be given to older children as a single dose at night (infants and young children metabolize the drugs quicker and the daily dose may have to be split into morning and evening portions to be effective for 24 hours).

References

1. Corbett, J. A. (1971). The nature of tics and Gilles de la Tourette's syndrome. *J. Psychosom. Res.*, **15,** 403–409
2. Dawson and Butterworth, K. (1979). Head banging in young children. *Practitioner*, **222,** 676–679
3. Nicol, A. R. (1982). Psychogenic abdominal pain in childhood. *Br. J. Hosp. Med.* **30,** 351–353
4. Hockaday, J. M. (1982). Headache in children. *Br. J. Hosp. Med.*, **30,** 383–391
5. Meadow, R. (1985). Management of Munchausen syndrome by proxy. *Arch. Dis. Child.*, **60,** 385–393
6. Dhillon, S., Ngwane, E. and Richens, A. (1982). Rectal absorption of diazepam in epileptic children. *Arch. Dis. Child.*, **57,** 264–267
7. Caufield, P. R., Caufield, C., Dooley, J. M., Tibbles, A. R., Fung, T. and Garner, B. (1985). Epilepsy after a first unprovoked seizure in childhood. *Neurology*, **35,** 1657–1666
8. Brown, J. K. and Sills, J. A. (1977). Status epilepticus. *J. Maternal Child Health*, **Oct,** 383–389
9. O'Donohoe, N. V. (1985). *Epilepsies of Childhood.* (London: Butterworths)

19

Normal variants

There are many conditions in children that are common, benign and, given time, self-correcting and can be termed 'normal variants'.

Their recognition and understanding are important if unnecessary treatment that is wasteful, unpleasant and even dangerous is to be avoided. Whilst the majority of these conditions can be observed and followed-up with 'masterly inactivity', blind unthinking underactivity has to be guarded against because of rare possibilities of serious conditions with similar symptoms and signs.

WHAT ARE THEY?

Normal variants represent the edges of the spectrum of child development.

Within every system there are broad *ranges of normality*. As a simple example the ranges of height and weight are wide and it would be foolish to assume without good reasons that children at upper and lower percentiles are abnormally short or tall or thin or fat. Age of first walking has a wide range of normality.

In addition there are conditions which are *abnormal* but which tend to *correct themselves* with time. Within this group are also those that may not completely resolve but which do no harm if left.

There is yet another group with accepted abnormalities but which are so widely prevalent as to be almost *inevitable stages of growing up*.

SIGNIFICANCE AND IMPORTANCE

Ranges of normality

The indices of normality have to be flexibly interpreted.

height

weight

physiognomy – take care not to label a child's facial appearance potentially abnormal until you have seen both parents.

shape of head

passing of developmental milestones depends on speed and normal children can travel at different rates.

Self-correcting abnormalities

Strawberry naevi

Strawberry naevi, even if large, have a strong tendency to disappear completely without scarring by the time the child is at primary school.

Umbilical herniae

In infants umbilical herniae disappear when the child begins to walk, but often some redundant skin remains that may need removal for cosmetic reasons later.

Non-retractile foreskins

These may not retract until the boy is 3–4 years old. That is normal. Forceful attempts at retraction cause trauma and scarring. There is no increased risk to balanitis or paraphimosis, provided that the foreskin is left alone.

Hydrocoele

This is common in male infants. They may be bilateral or unilateral. The infant scrotum normally is relatively much larger than at other stages of childhood. Given time most closed hydrocoeles will disperse within the first year. Surgical treatment may be necessary if the hydrocoele is so large that it interferes with normal hygiene or walking.

Undescended testes

No testis may be felt in an infant's scrotum. This may be a delay of normal descent and the boy should be re-examined every 6 months or so to assess progress. If the testes are not in the scrotum by the age of 2 years then possible surgery should be considered.

There is the opposite situation where both testes are felt in the scrotum at neonatal examination but 2 or 3 years later they become 'undescended' and are missing on examination. This may be temporary because of muscular contraction, but some of these remain undescended and require surgical orchidopexy.

Tongue tie

Tongue tie has not been proven to cause any difficulties with eating or talking. There are no good reasons for cutting the frenulum.

Orthopaedic conditions

There is a collection of orthopaedic conditions which fall into probable normal abnormalities, but with all these there may be need for treatment in a few cases where they are causing problems with function.

These are:

bow legs

knock knees

flat feet

curly small toes

over-riding 4th and 5th toes

intoeing gait (note that toe-walking may not be so innocent, as it may be a sign of a neurodevelopmental delay, in which case it is accompanied by other features such as late walking and late talking)

most clicking hips cease to click within a few weeks, but the possibility of CDH must be excluded if the click persists

Large tonsils and palpable cervical glands

These are present in all children between 3 and 8 years and are part of the catarrhal child syndrome (see p. 103).

Enuresis

Enuresis is a delay of normal automatic bladder control. Rarely is it associated with urinary tract infections and structural abnormalities but the possibility must be considered and excluded. Whether associated behavioural problems are cause or effect is arguable. It is more prevalent in social classes 4 and 5 and with poor housing and overcrowding.

Enuresis – % rates

Age	Boys	Girls
4–5	15%	10%
6–7	10%	8%
10	2%	2%

Soft cardiac murmurs

These may be heard in about one third of normal children. In very few is there any organic cardiac abnormality.

20

Accidents

Accidents are an inevitable part of childhood experience. Probably every child has at least one accident each year. Most accidents are minor but over 1000 children die each year from accidents in the UK.

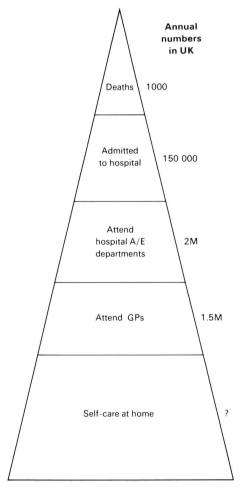

Figure 20.1 The accident iceberg (from reference 1).

There is an *iceberg* of severity of childhood accidents (Figure 20.1). In retrospect all accidents are preventable. The challenge is how they might be prevented in real life. It is useful to define at-risk groups and factors and to take preventive measures in individual cases.

DEATHS FROM ACCIDENTS

One third of all deaths in children in the UK are from accidents (Figure 20.2). These accident mortality rates in the UK are half those in USA and Canada[1].

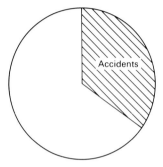

Figure 20.2 Deaths from accidents in children.

Motor vehicles are responsible for most accidents in children (Figure 20.3).

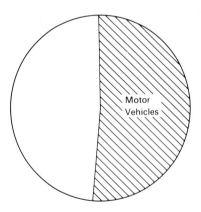

Figure 20.3 Causes of fatal accidents in children.

Causes of fatal accidents in children

	%
Motor vehicles	
(Pedestrians 35%)	
(Cyclists 10%)	
Drowning and suffocation	15
Burns/fires	10
Falls	5
Others	15
	100

The most prevalent injuries causing death are head injuries, respiratory obstruction and burns.

NON-FATAL ACCIDENTS

The annual number of childhood accidents is impossible to measure but it probably exceeds the total number of children.

The most frequent injuries are

cuts and bruises
burns (see Figure 20.4)
fractures and sprains

Where do they occur?

on roads	41%
at home	37%
falls from buildings and trees	7%
others	15%

Where in the home?

living room	30%
kitchen	18% (see Figure 20.5)
stairs	10%
bedroom	10%
hall	5%
bathroom–toilet	5%
around the home	20% ·
other	2%

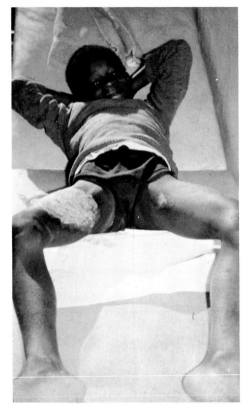

Figure 20.4 Winston was leap-frogging over a paraffin stove whilst his mother was out shopping.

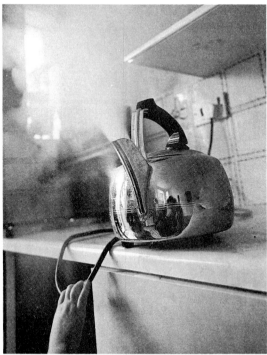

Figure 20.5 (From *Play it Safe*, Health Education Council and Scottish Health Education Group in association with BBC Television, by kind permission).

Accidents outside the home

more common in summer
more common in daylight
most in residential areas
small children on minor roads
older children on major roads
boys more than girls
cyclists are usually boys
high ride cycles are most dangerous
pedestrians – sudden 'dash across'
pedestrians – usually have accompanying adult

John bought his ice cream and dashed from behind a car. Fortunately, passing car going slowly, stopped in time to cause no injuries, but could have proved fatal.

At-risk groups

risks rise inversely with social class (i.e. much more class 5 than 1)
boys more than girls
boys more severely injured
higher rates in single-parent families
higher rates in larger families
higher rates when both parents at work
higher rates when children in care of older siblings

Medical students stood outside supermarkets and asked mothers where they kept dangerous objects, e.g. medicines, electric drills, paint stripper etc., and also found social class of head of household. 87% made *no* arrangement to keep things out of reach. Of 13% who did, only 2 were *not* social class 1, 2 or 3 (Pollak, personal communication).

WHAT CAN BE DONE

Use all opportunities to educate for prevention.

Children

small children must be protected
schoolchildren must be educated
adolescents must not take risks

Parents

Parents tend to be overconfident of their childrens' ability to take care of themselves. They need to be reminded and informed[2]. 'It will never happen to me'.

Home visits

Health visitors, nurses and doctors on home visits should point out obvious hazards and suggest preventive actions.

Community action

Joint actions by town planners, architects, doctors and the public should be taken to define hazards and to plan and act to prevent them. The benefits of car seat belts are an example of success.

References

1. OHE (1981). *Briefing No. 17 on 'Accidents'*. (London: Office of Health Economics)
2. Health Education Council (1981). *Play it Safe*. A Guide to Preventing Children's Accidents. (London: Health Education Council)

21

Non-accidental injuries

The exact incidence is unknown and frequency differs in different areas, 'inner cities' having the highest incidence.

For example, in *North Wiltshire* in 1972–3 Scott found a rate of 1 new case per 1000 children under 4 years[1]. On the other hand, in *Lambeth* during the same period of time, Kempe found a rate of 2 per 1000 under 3 years of age[2].

Many non-accidental injuries in young children are not seen and recorded by health professionals. This means that in the United Kingdom between 2000 and 5000 cases occur each year.

It seems that in a practice population of 2500 persons a general practitioner (family physician) can expect one case of non-accidental injury every 5–10 years. These numbers may not be large but the mortality rate is about 10% and a permanent serious damage rate in the child is 15%. Thus 1 in 4 abused children are killed or maimed, and a general practitioner may expect to see one death in his or her professional career.

Physical abuse of children has always existed and probably was submerged or accepted as a normal pattern of life. Gil believes that physical abuse of children is endemic in American society[3].

COMMON CHARACTERISTICS

The Parents

usually young
poor upbringing
often unmarried, living together or single parents
female-headed household – single, separated, divorced, widow
lower social groups with poor education and low income
poor marital and family relationships

151

may be a minority ethnic group
isolated with lack of support from family
bad housing, multi-occupiers, complaining neighbours
4+ children (all under 18 years)
unemployed fathers or father-equivalent[3]

There are differences in ethnic groups and customs in relation to attitudes to corporal punishment. Thus, American Indians never use physical force to discipline their children and have a very low rate of child abuse and non-accidental injuries. Black Americans and Puerto Ricans use physical force with high rates of non-accidental injuries.

'Father'

often not married to mother
personality problems
past history of violence
immature behaviour
alcoholic history
unemployed

(The following medical records illustrate how a family may present to their family practice.)

Medical Record

JOHNSON GEORGE
10 RYGATE ROW   D.O.B. 14.2.62.
BUILDERS LABOURER

Didn't go to work today. Says his back hurts. Wants a week off.

Lost his job. Living with Jean Brown who is due in 2 weeks

(Home visit)   Backache again. Wants a weeks off. ?Drinking too much.

Obviously rowing with Jean. He complains of her bad house-keeping and parenting skills. She is pregnant again.

Back with Jean again. In trouble with the police.
Wants a tonic.

Mother

neurotic and immature
unplanned and unwanted pregnancy

didn't 'bother' to organize an abortion

depressed after birth

poor antenatal attender

poor bonding with baby

frequent attender of clinics and surgeries often for inappropriate reasons

poor housekeeper, manager and disciplinarian

Medical Record

BROWN JEAN SHARON

10 RYGATE ROW   D.O.B. 5.10.64.

Missed period. Dare not tell mum (urged to do so). Living with George Johnson.

L.M.P. 24.12.81 resigned. A/N (Wants all A/N at hospital in case she sees mum in waiting room).
Delivery: N.D. 5.10. ?F.T. In S.C.N. 3 days. Doesn't want to breast feed. H/V to visit.

Failed P/N and family planning.

Pregnant again. Says George staying out late, very bad tempered.

A/N. N.A.D.

A/N. Hb.9 g. Double Fe. Smokes 15/day. 32 weeks. ?depressed.

Home in dreadful muddle. Wants housing letter.

George has left her.

George back. Feels can't cope with two children always whining and crying. H/V to visit.

Children

The children often fail to thrive following difficult births. There may be a large and disorganized family.

Mum complains that the abused child 'won't eat, won't sleep and is always whining and crying'. The child is often enuretic and clumsy with poor language development.

Although most child abuse leading to injuries occurs in the first year or two of life, it can occur at any age. Development is often delayed and handicap is present. There are signs of neglect.

Medical Record

BROWN JAMES
10 RYGATE ROW   D.O.B. 7.8.82.

Home visit	N.D. 5.10. Not feeding well. Exam. N.A.D. H.V.
Baby Clinic	Feeding better. Mum says cries a lot. 1st injection.
Baby Clinic	DNA 2nd injection.
Surgery	Mum says always miserable. Doesn't eat well. Nappy rash. Wheezy. ?gaining weight well. To come to Baby Clinic when better.
Baby Clinic	DNA
Surgery	Doesn't eat. Cries a lot at night. George gets cross. Wants a sedative.

Medical Record

BROWN SHARON
10 RYGATE ROW   D.O.B. 29.9.83.

Home visit	P/N.F.T, N.D.5.4. Feeding problems in hospital. Seems OK now.
Surgery	Mum says always whining and cries a lot. Never satisfied. Not a 'friendly' baby. (H.V. says home very disorganized, James always in pram, not cot.)
Baby Clinic	Ht. and Wt. at 3rd percentile. Head 25th.
Baby Clinic	DNA.
Surgery	URTI, irritable, 'won't sleep'.
Surgery	Chest N.A.D. but always 'miserable'.
Surgery	Brought by mum. Says James knocked her off the bed 2 days ago. Crying ever since. Thinks her left arm is 'funny'. O/E: ? left forearm. ?cigarette burn on left leg and bruising on buttock (Jean very defensive and anxious). →Hosp. (Phoned up houseman). Asked Jean to go with George to hospital – she says he is not home yet. Always 'out late'.

Grandmother

'chronic nerves'
poor relations with daughter
anxiety over grandchildren but no contacts

Medical Record

BROWN MARY
5 BROWNING HOUSE, SHELLY RD.   D.O.B. 7.7.36.

Worried about daughter. Jean always stays out late. 'Nerves' bad.

Depressed, tried to be reconciled with daughter but George J. very abusive. Jean sulky.

Sore throat. (Asked if Jean and baby OK.)

Flu, C.7. No contact with Jean. Would like to see her grandchild. (Doesn't know of second pregnancy.)

Depressed again. Worries about Jean and grandchildren

THE ABUSE

The child may present to the doctor with a quite unrelated presenting symptom. The child is often brought late in the incident. There is an improbable explanation for the injury. Bruises on the legs are explained as 'knocked legs on toy horse' *but* he had bruising of back too!
  Common injuries are:

bruising with finger and thumb marks of pinching and punching trauma, and tooth marks of biting

burns and scalds: note cigarette burns and note that scalds have sharply defined edges (Figures 21.1, 21.2)

displaced epiphyses with periosteal bruising and thickening

fractured skull

subdural haematoma

There may be 'frozen awareness' in the child – an expression and behaviour of apprehensive watchfulness. He cries if *anyone* approaches.

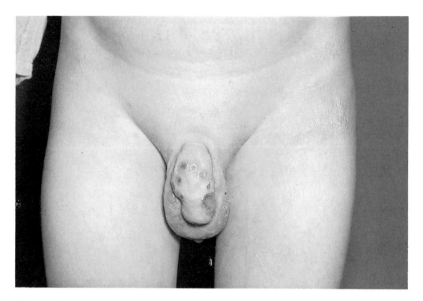

Figure 21.1 Non-accidental injury – penile burns produced by a cigarette (from Verbov and Morley, *Colour Atlas of Paediatric Dermatology*, p. 142, Lancaster: MTP Press, by kind permission).

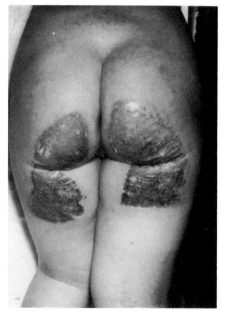

Figure 21.2 Burns from sitting on a hotplate (from Lissauer, *Paediatric Emergencies*, p. 257, Lancaster: MTP Press, by kind permission).

THE ABUSER

The most frequent abuser is the biological parent, *the mother*. Next comes the *stepfather* and *foster parents*. *Abusers* are usually of low educational and socioeconomic status. They deviate socially, emotionally, behaviourally and intellectually, and often belong to minority groups.

THE FAMILY DOCTOR

Although infrequent in a practice, child abuse is potentially fatal. Know your families and look for signs of neglect – unhappy or dirty child, and poor nutrition. Note 'at risk families' and alert the health visitor. Completely undress all suspicious cases and keep good notes. Refer suspicious cases to hospital for admission and speak to the paediatric resident.

References

1. Scott, P. D. (1973). Fatal battered baby cases. *Med. Sci. Law*, **13,** 197
2. Kempe, C. H. (1971). Paediatric implications of the battered baby syndrome. *Arch. Dis. Child.*, **46,** 28
3. Gil, D. G. (1978). In Lee, C. M. (ed.) *Child Abuse.* (Milton Keynes: Open University Press)

SECTION IV

Society, Family and Community

22

Problem families: children at risk

WHO ARE THE PROBLEM FAMILIES?

Are they problems to themselves, to their doctors and/or to society? Are they the 'fat folders' of the practice, always consulting for trivial worries and anxieties? Are they the 'thin folders,' seldom consulting, perhaps not even registered, not accepting preventive care, advice or help from what they see as authority?

PROBLEM FAMILIES HAVE DIFFERENT MEANINGS

To some they are the families who suffer several social disadvantages or deprivations, the effects of which may be compounded by an inability to cope with the everyday routine of living. To others a 'problem' family is a family in which at least one of the members has a personality or psychological 'problem' producing an adverse effect on other members and usually making medical management unsatisfactory.

Types of problem families

Social deprivation

   poor housing
   low social class
   low income
   many children
   unsupported mothers

Psychological problems

psychoneurosis
personality problems
psychosis
poor parenting skills
alcoholism, drug dependency, sexual perversion

Unable to cope

low budget, many mouths to feed
unstable family relations
resultant chaotic household and family life
no time or patience to cherish and care for children

Mixture of all three

How are they identified?

There are at-risk factors which are common and recurring in problem families

young, unsupported social class IV and V mothers
unplanned pregnancies
families of 4+ children
low income
poor housing
poor marital and family relations
parental neurosis
divorce and one-parent families
low parenting skills, low interest, love and care of children

These 'at-risk' factors have profound effects on the children in-volved.

Young, unsupported families, social class IV and V

higher infant mortality
lower birthweight
lower uptake of immunizations, etc. and preventive care
lower reading, spelling, writing and arithmetic skills
early school leaving
higher juvenile delinquency
poor housing
living in districts with fewer amenities

Unplanned pregnancies and 4 + children

birth hazards
low IQs
educational problems

Low income

poor housing
early school leaving
juvenile delinquency

Poor housing (see p. 217)

low income
fatherless families
sick or unemployed fathers
poor educational achievement
more often rehoused

Poor marital and family relations

behaviour problems in children
low discipline at home
lack of interest in school work
developmental delay, especially language
poor educational skills
family disruption
disorganized homes
juvenile delinquency

Parental neurosis

behaviour problems
emotional problems
neuroticism
delayed language development

Divorce and one-parent families

See pp. 167–72.

Low parenting skills and low interest, love and care of children

low sense of discipline
low sense of property and privacy
parental violence
poor school attainment
possible difficulty in forming relationships

Some children will suffer multiples of these factors and not all the effects can be attributed to one single factor.

HOW THE PRACTICE TEAM CAN HELP

Family doctors are well named: they deal with that bulwark of English society – the family. If one considers the effects which 'problem' families have upon the children of a practice, it is apparent that many children are 'at risk' of suffering either a handicapping condition or of failing to fulfil their potential in life. These risks might be seen as being due to circumstances in families, parents, children, housing, school and medical factors.

Family doctors and the other members of the practice team are well placed to define, study and relieve these social ills and their effects on children.

Every primary care team will have within it many of these 'problem' families. Naturally the number will be higher in 'inner city' districts, a factor not always recognized by the profession and health authorities. These families should figure prominently on the practice 'at-risk' registers. Their number will be higher than cases of cerebral palsy (one new case every 18 years); Down's syndrome (1 every 12 years); a blind child (1 every 45 years); and one severely deaf (1 every 50 years). The rewards of helping them will be greater and more immediate.

When to be aware of the problem families

The health visitor must give these families special care and attention.

The GP/health visitor must ensure that health and developmental surveillance is undertaken and defaulters followed up, and up and up assiduously.

Language development in particular needs testing.

The mother/child relationship should be observed and promoted.

PROVEN MEASURES

Work in Sheffield has shown that when health visitors give extra care and visits to 'risk' families, the level of child abuse is significantly reduced[1].

Mothers' groups, when child-rearing methods were discussed, have been shown to be helpful in reducing emotional problems.

An Israeli study has proved that children who received 'home stimulation' programmes in the first year of life were still at 9 years of age ahead in IQs and school achievement compared with controls[2].

An American study has shown the value of preschool help for 'deprived' children. When examined at 20 years of age and matched against a control group, such children were found to be holding down more good jobs, earning more money and were psychologically much more stable than the control group. The exercise showed how cost effective such preschool help had been[3].

Health visitors could be involved in a home stimulation programme – a Portage system for 'problem' families as well as for handicapped.

References

1. Sunderland, R. and Emery, J.L. (1979). Apparent disappearance of hypernatraemic dehydration from infants' death in Sheffield. *Br. Med. J.*, **2**, 575–576
2. Palti, H., Zilber, N. and Kark, S.L. (1982). A community-orientated early intervention programme integrated in a primary preventive child health service – evaluation of activities and effectiveness. *Community Health*, **4**, 202–314
3. Weikart, D.P., Bond, J.T. and McNeil, S.T. (1978). *The Ypsilanti Perry Preschool Project: Preschool Years and Longitudinal Results.* (London: High Scope Press Pub., National Children's Bureau)

23

Single (one) parent families

One-parent families make up 12% of all families and their proportions are increasing for a number of reasons:

changing social modes and customs with parents intentionally not marrying with a high risk of break-up of the union

more divorces and separations

NUMBERS AND RATES

In 1980 in the UK there were 1 million one-parent families and 1.6 million children involved[1]. 12% of all families are one-parent families[2]. Of these 10.5% are lone mothers and 1.5% are lone fathers (Figure 23.1).

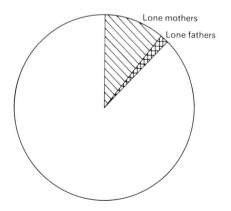

Figure 23.1 One-parent families.

Of the *lone mothers*, circumstances are (Figure 23.2):

single   21%
widows   16%
divorced   39%
separated   24%

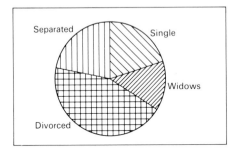

Figure 23.2   Lone mothers.

TRENDS

Numbers of one-parent families have more than doubled over 20 years[3] (Figure 23.3).

1961   474 000
1981   1 000 000

One-parent families create many difficulties for parents, children and society.

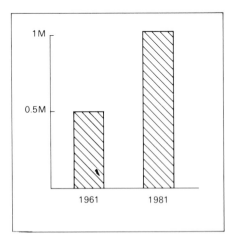

Figure 23.3   Numbers of one-parent families.

SOCIAL PROBLEMS

One-parent families are 58% of all families receiving *supplementary benefits*[1]. One-parent families are 51% of all families on *family income supplements*[1]. One-parent families are 52% of all families who have been *housed under 1977 Housing (homeless persons) Act*[1].

DISADVANTAGES FOR MOTHER

Particular problems and difficulties are[4]:

likely to be of *lower social class* with all the disadvantages

less likely subsequently to *marry*

likely to be *young teenager*

housing *inadequate*, council property with *lack of amenities* and *overcrowding*

frequent moves likely

less likely to receive early regular *antenatal care*

more likely to have *low haemoglobin in pregnancy*

more likely to *go out to work* when child is small

more likely to be a *heavy smoker*

likely to have *less money* than equivalent married or two-parent families.

DISADVANTAGES FOR CHILD

Compared with children of similar social class, legitimate or adopted, children in one-parent families:

lower *birth weights*

higher *perinatal mortality*

more likely to *die in first 5 years of life*

taken less often to *baby clinics*

suffer more *non-accidental injury*

attend hospital more often

suffer more *accidents*[4]

taken into care more often because of:

homelessness

illness of mother

mental disorder in mother

desertion

second or subsequent pregnancies[1]

More specifically, the children are more likely to suffer from *behavioural and developmental problems*, e.g.:

lower developmental achievement

more clumsy

poor speech development

more maladjustment

higher attendance rates at child guidance clinics[4]

Once they reach *school age* they have more problems:

attend less often

attend special schools more often

change schools more often

mothers less interested in child's school achievements

lower results in:
arithmetic
reading
draw-a-man scores
general knowledge

WHAT CAN THE PRIMARY CARE TEAM DO TO HELP?

(1) Develop *friendly and understanding relations* with young adult patients to encourage their attendance when in trouble.

(2) Encourage all members of the practice team (doctors, health visitors, practice nurses, school nurses) and others, such as teachers, to discuss *contraception* for young persons.

(3) Encourage youngsters to *prepare for marriage, and parenthood.*

(4) Offer advice and help to prevent further pregnancies until the family unit is stable.

(5) Use special doctor/patient relationship to encourage *early antenatal attendance* at practice or other clinics.

(6) Provide extra care and support during and after *pregnancy.*

(7) Encourage regular attendance at *baby clinic.*

(8) Be alert to *developmental and speech immaturity.*

(9) *Health visitors* have particular opportunities for long-term support (given the chance if they remain in area). They can encourage good child rearing and advise on the need for loving stimulation.

(10) *Social workers* can help with adequate housing, advice on financial and good housekeeping skills.

(11) The prime objective during infancy (and after) is to develop good *mothering and bonding.*

(12) Note that *adopted children* are less disadvantaged than one-parent children. The question of adoption may be appropriate.

ILLUSTRATIVE CASE (Figure 23.4)

This young girl appeared at her doctor's surgery, requesting that her illegitimate son should be taken into care. She had managed to bring him up well to date. She was handsome and athletic and an acrobat dancer in a circus. The manager had allowed her to have Jason with her up until now. Now that the circus was going on a European tour, he refused to let the boy go too. After much deliberation with the social workers, it was decided to foster him for the 3 months of the tour. (Her track record, as it were, was good.)

It proved to be a mistake. She never returned and could not be traced. So, Jason, who already lacked a father's love, now lacked a mother's too. In this case, there was a happy ending as Jason was a delightful boy and was later very successfully adopted.

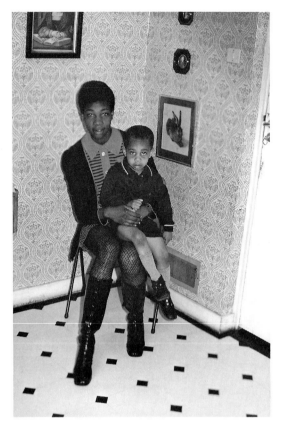

Figure 23.4

References

1. National Council for One Parent Families (1980). Report No. 5. (NCOPF)
2. GHS (1981). Government Household Survey (HMSO)
3. OPCS (1984). Office of Population Censuses & Survey (HMSO)
4. Crellin, E., Pringle, M. L. K. and West, P. (1971). *Born Illegitimate*. (Slough: NFEB for Childrens' Bureau)

24

Divorce and separation

We are now living in a high divorce society. Not only is divorce common, but remarriage also. Many of the practice's children are likely to spend much of their home life without one of their natural parents, often the father.

All studies demonstrate that children who can maintain good relationships with both parents will be better psychologically, emotionally and educationally than those who do not.

England is ranked 11th amongst 20 European countries for divorce rates, Hungary having the highest with East Germany and Denmark being second and third[1].

FACTS

1 in 3 of marriages ends in divorce

2 of 3 divorces involve children

For those parents who are under 20 the divorce rate is double that of those who are 20–25.

'Shot-gun marriages' because the girl is pregnant are a frequent reason for early marriage (under 20) and have high divorce rates.

The story of families 'A' and 'B' is horrific and confusing but not uncommon (see illustrative case).

Many workers are involved in care:

GP
receptionists
health visitors
social workers
school teachers

nurses
NSPCC
probation officer

Their efforts at prevention of future long-term behavioural problems are frustratingly minimal.

Divorce is increasingly common in early years of marriage when children are young.

1 in 3 of marriages now involves children who are young.

Divorce is more common in working classes.

50% of children of divorces have less contact with one parent after the divorce.

Children of divorces realize impermanence and instability for the first time. They do not like being left at school and insist on having a light left on at night. They may become angry and feel helpless and realize that their interests and those of the parents differ.

There may be aggression towards the remaining parent and siblings and there may be idealization of the absent parent.

Families 'A' and 'B'

Mr and Mrs A. were aged 32 and 35
They had four children aged 9, 8, 5 and 3½. There was great marital discord. Eventually, Mrs A. left home to live with her boyfriend. She took the two youngest with her. The 5-year-old girl had to change schools because of the move. The liaison lasted about 12 months and then she wanted to return to the marital home.

By this time Mr A. had a divorcee, Mrs B., living with him, the two older boys and the divorcee's own two boys who were aged 8 and 5.

Mr A. agreed to move out and live nearby in Mrs B.'s house.

Mrs A. returned, together with the two children. The 5-year-old now returned to her previous school, where she found Mrs B.'s 5-year-old. Mr and Mrs A.'s two older children refuse to visit their mother. Mrs B.'s 8-year-old is intensely jealous of Mr A.'s 8-year-old and they have had to move schools. Mr B. has access to his boys and this causes disharmony amongst them and the two older A. boys. To make matters worse, since they live very close to each other, the two families often meet, some of whom talk and some of whom do not.

Treating the behavioural symptoms of all (all are registered with the same family doctor) is a nightmare.

EFFECTS OF DIVORCE/SEPARATION

Ill effects differ with age. Older children may appear unaffected but their school work suffers.

Perinatal

Perinatal mortality rates are higher when the mother is unsupported at time of birth. This requires more care in antenatal and postnatal periods.

0–3 years

    regression of toilet training
    increased crying
    sleep problems
    temper tantrums
    social withdrawal

3–5 years

Half of the children show features of regression.

5–8 years

Depression manifests itself in different ways. They are withdrawn at home and excessively pre-occupied with events and people outside the home. They blame themselves for the divorce and have poor peer relationships.

Although these effects create major behavioural disturbances, with good care they can be minimized and most will have disappeared within 2–3 years.

Adolescents

They withdraw from in-family relationships and seek early heterosexual involvements.

Divorced parents (especially women) visit doctors more at time of separation with grief symptoms. Extra support should be provided for such divorcees and their children.

Custody of children after divorce

Custody is more often contested when divorce was on grounds of cruelty or unreasonable behaviour rather than adultery.

Three quarters of children were living with their mother when the divorce was filed.

One quarter of parents who had children with them were living temporarily with their own parents.

Regular access was exercised in 44%. Access was not exercised at all in 30%. Access was contested more often when father had custody[2].

Factors relating to after-effects

The after-effects depend on the relationship with the remaining parent. They usually last longer than 1 year. They are much better if relations are good with both parents.

Divorce often involves a move with loss of friends and neighbours as well as a parent. This also makes access by the other parent difficult.

Children of divorce suffer all the disadvantages of single-parent families and do less well than bereaved children.

There is no certainty that matters will be better if the parent re-marries.

Manipulation – involvement

Doctors, social workers and relatives may become emotionally entangled in inter-parent disputes. They may be manipulated by either or both parents.

The bitterness is such that the end results for the doctor may be complaints of serious professional misconduct by breaches of confidentiality. The doctor may be subpoenaed to give evidence in court actions between parents for custody of the child.

Divorce proceedings may be protracted, sometimes up to a year, and a decision about custody will take a similar time. This can create a bad situation for children who are left with one parent or a relative until the divorce becomes absolute and they then have to go either to the other parent or another relative.

A paediatrician was asked to see a 4-year-old girl Anna who was non-verbal. The child had a French father and an English mother and had lived in Switzerland. Mother and father were divorcing and mother had come, with Anna, to live in England with grand-mother.

Father and mother spoke French to each other, mother spoke English to Anna. In addition, mother was a career woman, out all day, and Anna had a succession of different speaking au pairs. No wonder she was non-verbal.

The paediatrician took Anna into a group for language-delayed children where she began to make progress, although it became obvious that the mother–child relationship was not good.

Soon the paediatrician was served an order to attend court. In court it became obvious that the mother was using Anna's need to receive language help as a reason for her living in England. The father, seen for the first time in court, obviously loved his daughter and was heartbroken by the decision of no access.

Anna's behaviour in the group was extremely disturbed for a long time afterwards (she had seen her father in court) and the mother removed her from the group and went to live in Scotland. It became obvious that the paediatrician had been used as a means of getting the child to England, away from her father.

WHAT CAN THE DOCTOR DO?

Anna's story is not unusual and it behoves the doctors involved to consider certain rules.

It is worth remembering that in any case of divorce the court must consider the children and a decree absolute is only granted when the judge is satisfied with the arrangements made for the children.

Whilst very difficult to achieve in practice, especially when both parents are family practice patients, the doctor should try not to be drawn into taking 'sides'. Anna's case shows how this is not in the child's best interests.

If it is known that parents are likely to divorce, the family doctor, whilst remaining neutral, can offer counselling even if the marriage ends in divorce. This is worthwhile because what is best for the children can be discussed, and the idea of regular access aired. So often one party objects to this, and tries to influence the child against the other party. It has been known for children, who initially refused to visit one parent, to eventually over-react in later life by unjustifiably rejecting totally the parent with whom they were first living.

Those in contact with the children of recently divorced parents should remember that to some children it is as bad or worse than a bereavement and that time needs to pass for recovery.

References

1. Gibson, C. (1974). *Br. J. Sociol.*, **25,** 79
2. Quoted in: Gibson, C. (1973). Social trends in divorce. *New Society*, 5 July, 6–8
3. *United Nations Demographic yearbook* (1978)
4. Eekalaar, J. and Clive, E. (1977). Children in divorce. *New Society*, 19 May, 344
5. Richards, M. P. M. and Dyson, M. (1982). *Separation, Divorce and Development and Children; A Review.* Unpublished report of DHSS (London)
6. Richards, M. P. M. (1984). Children and divorce. In Macfarlane (ed.), *Progress in Child Health*, Vol. 1. (Edinburgh: Churchill-Livingstone)

25

Children in care

In 1982 7.5 per 1000 children under 18 were 'in care' of local authority social services departments[1]. This means:

1 child in 130 in care
3–4 children per GP in care
12–15 children per group practice in care

The total number of children in care in Great Britain and rates per 1000 children in 1961–1982 were[2]:

	1961	1971	1976	1980	1981	1982
Number in care (000)	72	102	118	117	114	109
per 1000 population under 18	6.0	6.4	7.5	7.8	7.7	7.5

Although numbers are falling, so are the numbers of children under 18, so the rates remain constant.

Local authorities have responsibilities to provide a care service to families (i.e. voluntary) in certain circumstances:

(1) Parents are ill, physically or mentally, and unable to care for the child. May be temporary or longer.

(2) Child is an orphan or has been abandoned.

(3) Child has committed a criminal offence.

(4) When the child is receiving 'no proper care and attention' and it is in the best interests of the child to be removed.

(5) If a child is to be adopted and afterwards.

The 1975 Children's Act emphasized that the welfare of the child was of major concern.

Children may be taken into care in a variety of ways.

Voluntary

This means it happens with the consent of the parents, in which case the parents can take the child back at any time within 6 months of the beginning of care. After 6 months, 28 days notice must be given to the local authority.

Compulsory Care Order

This is much more difficult to achieve. When granted the local authority has full supervision over the child until he/she is 18.

A Safety Order

This lasts for 28 days and is made by a magistrate who is satisfied that there is a need for care and the parents refuse voluntary admission of the child 'to a place of safety'. Anyone can apply at any time, but, in practice, usually a social worker or an officer of the NSPCC applies. After 28 days, the Safety Order cannot be renewed.

An Interim Care Order

This is sometimes made, for a further 28 days, particularly if the social workers are unprepared for a full court hearing for a compulsory Care Order.

Care Order

A Care Order is more difficult to achieve and follows care proceedings. If the court grants this, the local authority has full supervision of the child until he/she is 18.

A Supervision Order

This can be made for 3 years – or until the child is 18 years old. In these cases the child remains at home but the parents have a 'contract' with either a social worker or a probation officer who will oversee the welfare of the child. Very often, in those cases where an application for a discharge of a Care Order has been successful, a Supervision Order may be made.

Wardships

Wardships are made by the High Court and the custody of the child remains with the Court, which becomes the child's guardian. Although anyone can make an application to the Court, expenses are incurred which the applicant may have to bear.

WHY IN CARE?

The most frequent reasons for children being placed into care are:

neglect and ill treatment
guilty of an offence
deserted by parent(s), other parent unable to provide care
unsatisfactory home conditions
not receiving adequate education
matrimonial (parents) causes
long-term illness of parent(s)
short-term illness of parent
beyond parental control

AGES

Children of all ages are taken into care but the likelihood increases with age (Figure 25.1) The highest rates are in the 10–14 quinquennium. This is because it is at this time that children tend to commit offences as well as being exposed to other reasons for being taken into care.

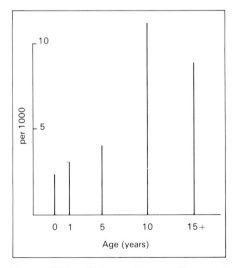

Figure 25.1 Children in care (from reference 11).

WHERE ARE THEY?

The manner of accommodation of children in care shows that 1 in 5 of the children are living with their natural parents, a guardian, relative or friend. Of the others almost one half are boarded out with foster parents.

The table shows the trend away from residential care towards boarding out with foster parents.

Place of children in care

	1977 (%)	1982 (%)
Boarded out	34	42
Local authority homes	33	27
Voluntary sector homes	4	3
Under charge of parent, guardian, relative or friend	18	19
Other accommodation	11	9

Children's Homes

There are three types of homes:

Large homes (over 50 children) where the children are grouped into small units. (The most seriously disturbed children are in such homes.)

Grouped cottages with 8–20 children per cottage. Each unit is self-contained with its own facilities, such as recreation hall and sick bay.

Family groups, each with 6–10 children. Each group is run by a housemother, who may have children of her own and whose husband follows his own occupation.

Children under 5 tend to be housed in residential nurseries or voluntary houses (? foster homes). Children needing short-term care are looked after in reception centres. These centres also serve as assessment units for children needing long-term care. About one half of residential staff are untrained.

WHO GOES INTO CARE?

The National Child Development Study reported characteristics of children likely to be taken into care[3].

working class (social classes IV and V)
crowded homes
homes with few amenities
more siblings than average
frequent house and school moves
illegitimate
young mothers
early gestation, low birthweight and small stature
lower weight and height (than average)
more clumsy
school reports 'scruffy, underfed and unattractive'
learning and behaviour problems
poor language range
poor reading
less general knowledge
lower IQs

These are, of course, just the children who are already at risk of not fulfilling their potential, so that a very heavy responsibility rests on local authorities and social workers to ensure that these children have as stable and loving a background as possible. It is often impossible to achieve this ideal.

MacAllister and Mason[4] studied the relationship between settings for juvenile delinquency and for children being taken into care. The Children's and Young Persons Act 1969 assumed that similar factors were involved. However, whilst it was clear that child density factors, unemployment, overcrowding, etc. were common to both, taking children into care was more associated with unemployment and low income; juvenile delinquency was more highly associated with overcrowding, high birth rate and poor housing. This research suggests that 'personal space' might be more important in delinquency, whilst economic factors are more important in a child being taken into care.

WHAT OUTCOMES?

Of those who spend 6 months in care 80% are likely to remain in care until the age of 18[5]. This study found for children in care:

50% of children in care aged 5-11 had been in care for more than 4 years

80% had been admitted before the age of 5

50% had been admitted before the age of 2

76% had no, or very infrequent, contact with either parent

17% in long-term care required 'substitute parents'

EFFECTS OF BEING IN CARE

Children are already disadvantaged when taken into care. Therefore, it is important to ensure extra good care to prevent ill effects of separation and rejection. Those in long-term care who do not receive care, affection and bonding tend to have difficulties in human relationships when adult. These children are prone to behaviour problems and are below average in intelligence[6]. Such problems make good fostering difficult.

Theories behind taking children into care have changed over the years. Earlier, many workers had taken to heart the importance of an early, secure environment and the development of attachment and the general policy was to keep children at home with mum under almost all circumstances. It was also modish to think that the mother had needs too and having her child at home with her was helpful to her maternal feelings.

Furthermore, sometimes it was thought that when a child was taken into care, especially to a foster home, a complete break with parents was best.

With time, it has become clear that home is not best under *all* circumstances. Sometimes psychological and physical violence make home unsafe. However, it is clear that those who have to make this decision with its inherent responsibility, have an awesome task. Nowadays, children and their needs are given much higher priority compared with their parents. It is also recognized that most research shows that keeping some link with the parents is beneficial to children and is to be encouraged.

The type of care affects outcome. Adopted children do well and compare equally with peers of natural parents[7] and fostering[8].

Homes

Working in the 1960s, the late Professor Jack Tizard showed, without doubt, that residential care for children did not depend only on available money and adequate staff, but depended also on the amount of interaction which took place between the children and the staff. He also found that hostel units gave better care to children compared with hospital units with at least an equivalent staff ratio[9].

Good outcomes of care for chronic handicaps, whatever the medical, nursing and physical care necessary, depend on love, security and stimulation, as in all children.

ILLUSTRATIVE CASES

Mr T. and Miss W. were both heroin addicts. Miss W. gave birth to James in hospital. He suffered from withdrawal symptoms soon after birth, but recovered. Miss W. refused to take him 'home' because it was unsuitable (one filthy room). He was taken into care. He went to a local authority nursery and after 9 months, Miss W. began to visit him. When he was 1 year old, she asked to have him with her since she and Mr T. were re-united after a separation. James, who was showing developmental delay, went 'home'. Although both undergoing treatment, Mr T. and Miss W. were still addicted.

Approximately 7 months later, the police were called to James' home by neighbours, where they found James lying on a bed, with a syringe hanging from his upper arm. He was again in care for 2 years. Miss W. was now living alone, but 'improved'. She wanted James back again. He went. He continued 'to and fro' twice more, until the local authority eventually took him into long-term fostering. He is mentally retarded, has partial sight, is underweight and has small stature.

Mrs M. was aged 60, a widow. She had two sons, but was sad that she had no grandchildren. Both sons, although married for several years were childless. One son and his wife had tried to adopt for 3 years. When they had almost given up hope of ever being offered a baby for adoption, the social services suddenly asked them if they would take a brother and sister aged 4 and $2\frac{1}{2}$ years. They had both been the subject of child abuse and the girl had been badly burned and required a series of operations for skin grafting. They were delighted and their entrance into her life transformed Mrs M. She was busy baby sitting, visiting, buying clothes and presents, her depression forgotten.

The children settled in well, but when after 6 months, the adoption case came to court, the mother suddenly refused to give consent. However, after a delay of another 6 months, the adoption went ahead. When the girl had her next skin-grafting, the nursing staff all mentioned her changed behaviour whilst in hospital. She was a model patient, although when admitted previously, whilst in care, she had been extremely difficult to manage. The boy had his neglected squint dealt with and both are now happy children attending normal schools.

WHAT CAN THE DOCTOR DO?

He probably cannot do very much but be aware of the problems of children in care in his practice. They should receive even more kindness and consideration than others.

GPs associated with children's homes and with foster parents should strive to emphasize *caring* as well as *training*.

They should make efforts to overcome natural reluctance to attend *case conferences* because they may lead to children being taken into care. The family doctor probably knows more about the family background than others at the conference. His/her views may affect the future course of the child's life.

Children have rights and needs as well as parents. They may not have an adult voice to represent them.

References

1. Knapp, M. (1985). *Nuffield/York Portfolio No. 7.* (London: Nuffield Provincial Hospitals Trust)
2. Social Trends 15 (1985). Children in care of local authority by type of accommodation and age group. Table 7.34, p. 120. (HMSO)
3. Mapstone, E. (1969). Children in care. *Concern, J. Nat. Child. Bureau,* **3,** 23
4. MacAllister, J. and Mason, A. (1972). Child delinquency and child care. *J. Criminol.,* **12,** 280
5. Rowe, J. and Lamber, L. (1973). *Children who Wait: a Study of Children Needing Substitute Parents.* (Association of British Adoption Agencies)
6. Pringle, M. K. (1974). *The Needs of Children.* (London: Hutchinson)
7. Seglaw, J., Pringle, M. I., and Wedge, P. (1972). *Growing up Adopted.* (Slough: National Foundation for Educational Research/National Children's Bureau Report)
8. McKay, M. L. (1980). Planning for permanent placement. *Adoption and Fostering,* **4,** 19
9. Tizard, J. (1964). *Community Services for Mentally Handicapped.* (London: Oxford University Press)
10. DHSS (1984). *Children in Care in England and Wales 1982.* (HMSO)
11. *Children Today* (1986), p. 14 (NCH)

26

Like mother, like child – keeping it in the family

No branch of medicine, save family medicine, has the privilege of feeling a baby *in utero*, perhaps seeing the baby being born, caring for the baby during infancy, childhood and adolescence and, later, feeling *in utero* the next generation.

Family doctors are, therefore, well placed not only to study the natural history of disease, but also the study of illness and disease in families and over two or, sometimes, three generations.

'*Keeping it in the family*' might be subdivided into:

inherited disease
familial disease
problems due to family conditions (it is with this group that we are mainly concerned)

INHERITED DISEASE

Congenital malformations may be attributable to *genetic* or *environmental* factors interacting in the intrauterine environment.

Some *purely environmental* factors have been defined as in the rubella syndrome, cytomegalovirus disease and the foetal alcohol syndrome.

Paediatrics has progressed so that much more detail is available regarding *genetic inheritance*.

The *whole* chromosome may be involved – as in Down's syndrome and Turner's syndrome.

Or there may be *gene mutation*, divided into:

Homozygous   Huntington's chorea
Marfan's syndrome

Heterozygous   Congenital deafness
Ichthyosis congenita

The importance for the generalist must be to take note of any consanguinity, abnormal family history and detailed perinatal history.

FAMILIAL DISEASE

Familial is defined as occurring in or affecting different members of the same family, possibly because science has not yet discovered the exact abnormality or factor.

Conditions in which a family history is prominent:

retinitis pigmentosa
dyslexia
shuffling
congenital dislocation of the hip
pyloric stenosis
cleft palate

PROBLEMS DUE TO FAMILY CONDITIONS

Intergeneration factors are related to parenting skills marital discord, child battering, illegitimacy and child rearing practices. There are other examples:

Children with many siblings are more likely to have large families themselves[1].

Children whose later marriage ends in divorce are more likely than those who do not divorce to have suffered from parental discord and separation[2].

There may be a three generation pattern – grandparents have a poor marriage, parents suffer marital discord and separation and and the child divorces.

A new mother who has experienced early childhood separation and discord is more likely, than a child who did not, to have poor early mothering skills and a baby with more problems[3, 4].

Illegitimate children are more likely to produce illegitimate children themselves[5].

Girls with teenage pregnancies are more likely to come from a one-parent family, unsupported and to have experienced parental marital discord and separation[6].

Parents who batter their children are likely themselves to have come from a home with marital disharmony and trauma, often 'broken' homes[7].

When parents separate, their children are more likely than those whose parents do not separate to conceive outside marriage and to have their first child before they are 20 years old[8].

Family 'B': Father came to consult with a sore throat. The throat was inflamed. He was not given an antibiotic.

Three days later, mother brought the daughter, aged 4 years, to the surgery. Although she appeared to be quite well, she had a peeling skin rash on both palms. Slight peeling was also found on both soles of the feet. She did not have a sore throat, nor was she willing to accept having had one in the immediate past weeks. She was not given any treatment.

Two weeks later, a house call was requested to the son, aged 9, who was ill in bed. He was feverish, ill with a swollen and tender left elbow joint. He was prescribed salicylates and the next day was still ill, feverish but the elbow was now better, but his left knee was now swollen and painful. A consultant paediatrician's opinion was sought and the diagnosis of rheumatic fever made. Terry developed a soft diastolic murmur. Serial ECGs were always negative.

Did they all have a streptococcus?

Family 'W': Mrs W. was always coming to the surgery. She suffered from migraine. No treatment ever made it better. Her facies was anxiety personified. No real cause for her anxiety was ever unfolded.

Later, she began bringing her son with vague headaches and ill-defined abdominal pains. Brian was following in mother's footsteps.

One day a request was made for a home visit. Brian's pains were so bad he was confined to bed. There were no signs of an acute abdomen. There were signs, however, of Mrs W's anxiety. Not only the carpet, but most of the furniture of the sitting room was shrouded in polythene. Nothing could portray this mother's obsessional anxiety so poignantly as the polythene. Not surprisingly, Mr W., a small, quiet man, spent most of the evenings 'out'.

Spoilt girl syndrome: Not common but easily recognizable when present. Only child with elderly parents. Lives in a financially up-wardly mobile home. Had every conceivable status-seeking toy when little. Always wears beautiful clothes. Both parents 'adore' her, especially dad. Leaves school at 16 for a 'nice' job, e.g. secretary or shop assistant in 'good' shop. Suffers from dysmenorrhoea, migraine, mild anxiety symptoms. Spends long time in her own room playing records. Few friends (Mum and Dad enough).

Marries a handsome, slightly socially inferior young man with prospects. At the wedding, both parents thought she looked beautiful. Son-in-law hardly mentioned.

Now living in a well-furnished flat, mostly bought by her parents. After not being able to 'manage' the pill, she becomes pregnant. Forceps delivery for long labour. It is described, even after months, as 'agony'. She will 'never have another child'.

Nowadays, she spends a great deal of time 'round at mum's'. Her little girl, beautifully dressed, with many large toys, is now the 'apple of her grandparents' eye'.

The marriage is not going well. She complains of frigidity. He complains 'she is always round at mum's'. She dislikes her in-laws. Her daughter is likely to follow the same pattern as her mother.

Family 'C': This attractive mother with her handsome family might appear to have no problems (Figure 26.1). But this is not the case.

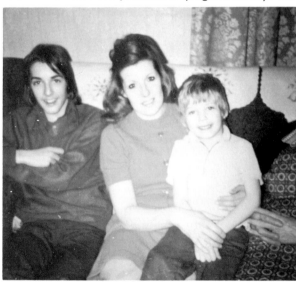

Figure 26.1

192

Mrs C. has brought her son to the doctor because he is not able to read or spell. He is 9 years old (Figure 26.2), was very depressed when father died suddenly (see later) and spent 18 months in a Child Psychiatry Unit. Mrs C. herself attends her family doctor frequently for depression and insomnia. She is unhappily married and thinking of leaving her husband, but does not know how to keep the family home going if she does so.

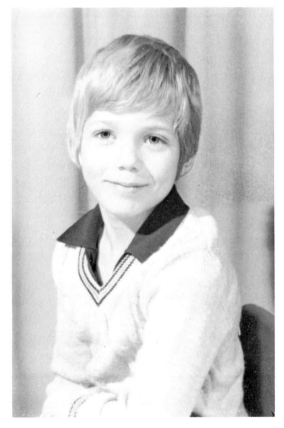

Figure 26.2

Mr C. is an alcoholic (Figure 26.3). He has suffered from oeso-phageal varices and shows the abdominal scar of a portacaval shunt done as a last resort to stop his uncontrollable bleeding of 30 pints of blood. Mr C. later died, following a cerebral haemor-rhage. Postmortem showed effects of alcoholic cirrhosis.

At the same time as Mr C. was recuperating from his operation, Mrs C's father was lying upstairs in the same house in the final phases of liver failure due to long-standing alcoholism. He had ascites (Figures 26.4 and 26.5).

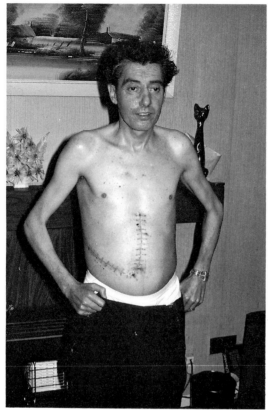

Figure 26.3

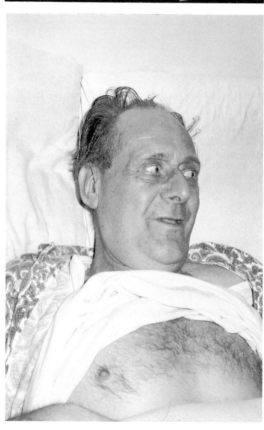

Figure 26.4

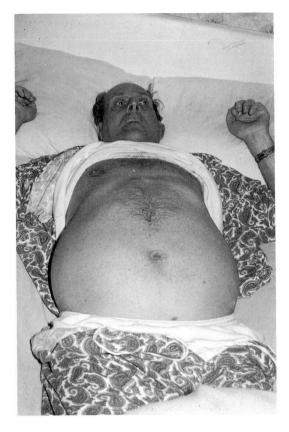

Figure 26.5

Alcohol weaved a fatal thread through three generations of a family all sharing one home.

Children of alcoholics have similar characteristics:

Girls

Love mother, hate father, or vice versa, feel rejected when father drinks.
Often pessimistic, withdrawn, very vulnerable when grown up.
Suffer anxiety, depression, temper tantrums and nocturnal enuresis when young.

Boys

Feel confused, have unpredictable relationship with parents.
May have disturbed relationship with non-drinking parent
Find difficulty in making friends, social isolation.
May be revengeful or afraid of alcoholic parent.

195

May turn against both parents.
Homosexuality is more likely.

Both sexes are more likely, themselves, to become alcoholic than children whose parents are not alcoholic.

Family 'K': Mr K. was from Mauritius. He was a skilled electrician but in harsh immigrant conditions could not obtain a job commensurate with his skills. He was doing much overtime in a menial job. Even this barely paid for the rent of the miserable one room in which he, his wife and son, Paul, were living.

He found relief by joining his mates in the pub. His pretty wife, from Cyprus, spent long hours alone in the one room, with Paul, awaiting her husband's return.

The family joined a new family doctor's group practice. The new doctor looked at Mrs K. who had brought Paul for intractable eczema. He had attended many skin departments, had many lotions and potions, nothing helped.

Why was Mrs K. so severe with her son? Her reactive depression was caused by her husband's late evenings and also because he started to beat her sometimes when he had had 'too much' to drink. She in turn felt stern and annoyed with Paul who was always scratching and often fractious. Paul took his grouse out on his skin.

The pecking order was: the father, disgruntled with society, took 'it' out on his wife; his wife, depressed with her harsh life, took 'it' out on her son; and the son, itching and irritable, took 'it' out on his skin.

References

1. Berent, J. (1953). 'Relationship between family size of two successive generations. *Millbank Mem. Fund. Quart.*, **31**, 39–50
2. Langer, T. S. and Michael, S. T. (1963). *Life Stress and Mental Health.* (Collier Macmillan)
3. Frommer, E. and O'Shea, G. (1973). Antenatal identification of women liable to have problems in managing their infants. *Br. J. Psychiat.*, **123**, 149–156
4. Frommer, E. and O'Shea, G. (1973). The importance of childhood experience in relation to problems of marriage and family building. *Br. J. Psychiat.*, **123**, 157–160
5. Crellin, E., Pringle, M. L. K. and West, P. (1971). *Born Illegitimate, Social and Educational Implications*, (Slough: NFER)
6. Wolkind, S. N. and Kruk, S. (1985). Teenage pregnancy and motherhood. *J. R. Soc. Med.*, **78**, 112–116

7. Oliver, J. E. and Taylor, A. (1971). Five generations of ill treated children in one family pedigree. *Br. J. Psychiat.*, **119,** 473–480
8. Illsley, R. and Thompson, B. (1961). Women from broken homes. *Sociol. Rev.*, **9,** 27–54

27

Cultural patterns

Cultural mores have more effect on parents and their children than is generally supposed. Differing child rearing practices are often due to differing cultural patterns, and produce differing patterns of development (Figures 27.1 and 27.2). Margaret Mead put it well – 'The child will have, as an adult, the imprint of his culture upon him, whether

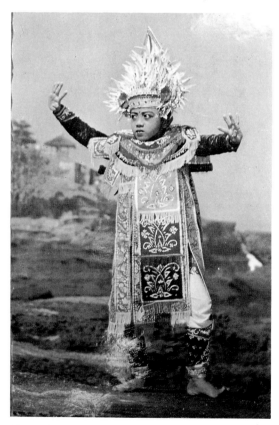

Figure 27.1 Nepalese dancer.

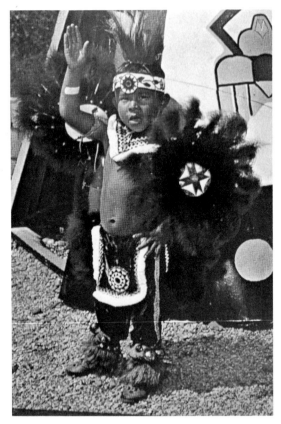

Figure 27.2   Cherokee Indian.

society hands the tradition with a shrug, throws it to him as a bone
to a dog, teaches him each time with care and anxiety, or leads him
to manhood as if he were on a sightseeing tour – but, whichever
method his society chooses will have far-reaching results in the attitudes of the growing child, upon the way in which he phrases the
process of growing up, and upon the resentment or enthusiasm with
which he meets the inevitable social pressures from the adult world'[1].

The point is illustrated by contrasting two differing cultures, the
difference between a child in Juxtlahuaca, Mexico and a Manus child,
Admiralty Islands, New Guinea.

The *Mexican* cultural pattern is of a close communal life, no private
property, individual's wishes subordinated to the welfare and har-
mony of the 'barrio'. The baby is subject to the 'Evil Eye' and is
protected by living on mother's back until weaned at 18 months. He
then has to learn by imitation of an elder sibling, who is now in charge

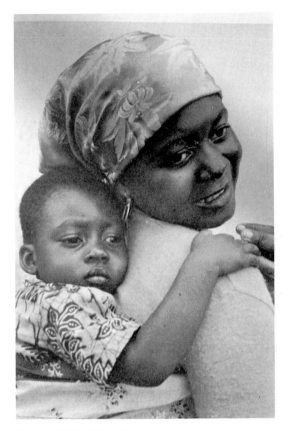

Figure 27.3 New Guinea.

of the child. By the age of 6 years, the age of reason is attained and the child is expected to undertake many adult household chores. Fighting is forbidden, children are not allowed to play with each other and become adult members of society early, although gradually.

In contrast the *New Guinea* cultural pattern is of parents whose marriage was arranged. The parents live with the father-in-law. The wife must not be seen by her father-in-law, or brothers-in-law, who also live in the house. Life is separate and in a small unit, although the bond between father and son is stronger than between husband and wife. The baby lies along the nape of his mother's neck (Figure 27.3) and goes everywhere with her. By three, he is expected to swim, dive and climb trees. The child must have a high respect for property, perfect control of his body and know his place in the seasonal rituals which play such a big part in his life. On the other hand, he is taught no self-control, no respect for elders, no discipline.

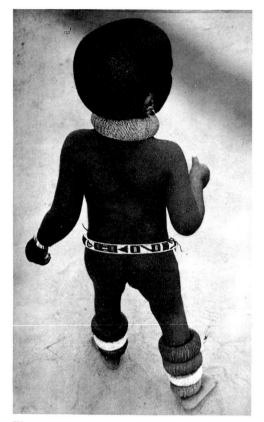

Figure 27.4

The children of New Guinea are renowned for their magnificent physique and athletic power (Figure 27.4). They have no self-discipline, intellectual thought, respect for property or age.

The Mexican children grow up to be timid and passive. They are introspective, withdrawn and suspicious, with little value of the individual but a high respect for age.

HISTORICAL TRENDS

Cultural attitudes towards children have changed over the centuries. Initially, babies and children were disregarded and only slowly, from the Middle Ages onwards, childhood gradually became accepted as a part of man's development. By the 20th century, Freud was saying that 'the child is father of the man'. Thus *Egyptian culture* believed that the first-born child should be sacrificed to the gods. The *Romans* thought it wise to kill the children of their enemies.

The Middle Ages, when perinatal mortality was high, had many folklores to ward off evil spirits to give the baby long and healthy life, such as:

wearing coral was thought to ward off fits (Figure 27.5)

a passing beggar was called in to become a godparent (Elizabethan England)

regular enemas kept the child in good health (17th century France)

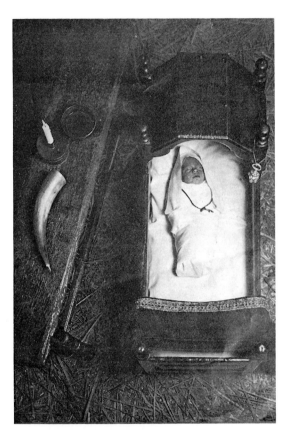

Figure 27.5 Swaddled baby wearing coral necklet.

Swaddling, which was a widespread practice in the world in the Middle Ages (Figure 27.5), has been shown[2] to produce passive children with hypersomnia, bradycardia, schizoid features and late walking[3]. Dislocation of the hips is also said to have been more frequent.

The aristocracy in England have a long tradition of separation of mother and child, with first the wet nurse (Figure 27.6), later apprenticeship with a noble family and, nowadays, boarding school.

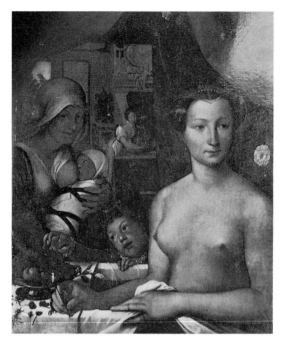

Figure 27.6 Gabrille d'Estrées, favourite of Henri IV, and her baby at the breast of a wet nurse.

That different cultures have different experiences and interpretations is well illustrated by the fact that Eskimos have 16 different words for snow[4], yet, when I was using a snowstorm under a glass case to test visual fields in a Nigerian boy, he asked 'What's that?' and then asked 'What is snow?'.

MULTIRACIAL UK

The United Kingdom is now a multiracial society, with many differing cultural patterns (Figure 27.7). In 1977, people of New Commonwealth and Pakistani ethnic groups (NCWP) origin represented 3.4% of the population. It includes those born in NCWP but not of UK origin, their descendants born in the UK. It includes those born in Cyprus, people of mixed descent but not coloured people of South Africa or USA.

Figure 27.8 illustrates the youth of the immigrants. Figure 27.9 shows striking differences in the conditions of birth of the nation as a whole, West Indian and Indian subcontinent births.

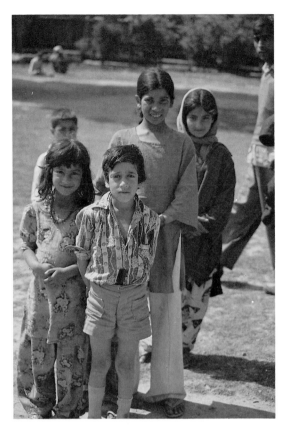

Figure 27.7   Muslim girl wearing special trouser suit.

The cultural patterns of the immigrants from the Indian subcontinent, the West Indies and Africa differ much in their family lives and child rearing practices.

Some characteristics of patterns on the Indian subcontinent

Often an arranged marriage
Father is head of household
Tightly knit family life
Many relatives living in UK
Young married couples often live with parents
The family 'dreams of returning home'
Mothers more often stay at home
Their English is poor or non-existent

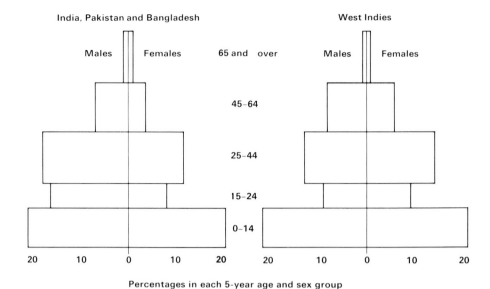

Figure 27.8 Age and sex structure of populations originating from India, Pakistan, and Bangladesh, and from the West Indies, 1976[8].

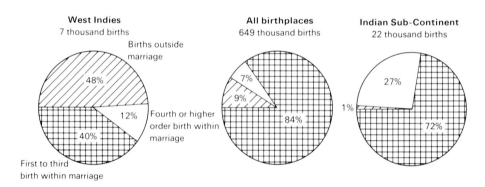

Figure 27.9 Births by birthplace of mother, 1976[8].

Muslims prefer wives to be looked after by woman doctor
Often illiterate
Prefer to keep child minding arrangements within the culture
In UK usually bottle feed their babies
Wean babies late
Babies tend to be small in weight at birth
High stillbirth and perinatal mortality
High rates of handicap
Schoolchildren have problems with diets, fasting and clothes and
   swimming

African cultural patterns

Parents usually married before arrival in UK

They intend to stay 'temporarily'

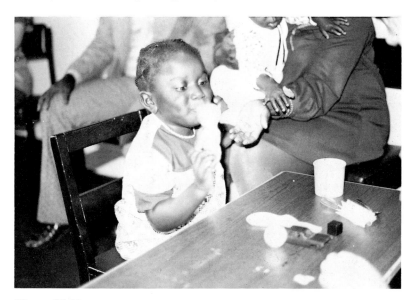

Figure 27.10

Although they speak their own patois, their command of English is usually good

The married couple tend to come from wealthy cultivated homes

Father is head of the household

The mother usually goes out to work, in a menial job, whilst father is studying for a degree or other skills

Usually few relatives in UK

Children are often fostered with Caucasian for preference, and may be seen by parents rather infrequently

Children – or whole family – often return to Africa for several months' holiday

Many children are bottle fed. They are weaned late

Iron deficiency anaemia is common at weaning time

Sickle cell trait occurs in 20–40% of Africans

West Indian cultural patterns

Usually marry in UK

Matriarchal society

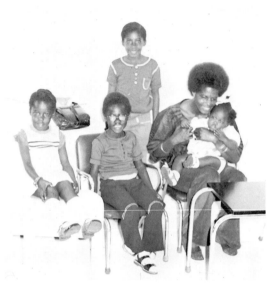

Figure 27.11

No settled family life

Many stepfathers and stepsiblings in family unit

Mothers out at work, usually full-time

Good basic English

Here to stay

Accepting of English educational system, but often unofficial child minders because nursery places hard to find

Mothers are too busy to play with their children

Mostly in social classes 4 and 5

Few grandparents living near[5]

Higher rates in care

Babies are usually breast and bottle fed (breast at night)

Early weaning

Children have a high incidence of behaviour problems[6], developmental and educational delay[5, 7] and schoolgirl pregnancies[5]

Sickle cell trait occurs in 10% of the West Indian immigrants

Special problems due to cultural patterns

Asian babies have a high rate of stillbirth, congenital malformations and infant mortality. These are possibly due to poor antenatal care, poor diet and/or intermarriages and late booking for care.

Mortality rates of babies born to mothers from Pakistan after the first weeks of life are over twice the level for babies of mothers born in the UK (Figure 27.12).

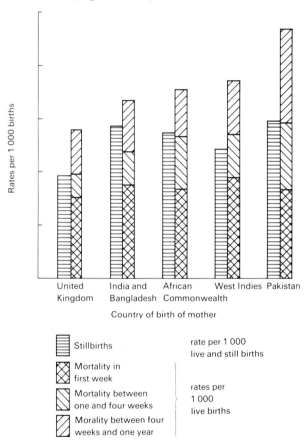

Figure 27.12 England and Wales stillbirth and mortality rates in the first year of life 1975–77, by country of birth of mother. Source: Studies in medical and population subjects, 41. HMSO, 1980.

The lower educational achievement of the West Indian child-ren[5, 9, 10] leads to a higher level of unemployment of West Indian school leavers and juvenile delinquency[11].

Adolescence appears to be a period of stress for Asian children, especially girls. They are brought up in two cultures, one at home and one at school. The Asian family more than any other immigrant group views with horror their children marrying outside their ethnic group. The adolescents are pulled by two different cultures.

HEALTH PROBLEMS

West Indian children, living in London[5] have been found to suffer more than the indigenous population from:

infantile eczema
otitis media
asthma
hay fever
nocturnal enuresis
chilblains
burns and accidents
withdrawn behaviour
conduct disorder (boys)[6]

Asian children have higher degrees of:

URTI
childhood fevers
iron deficiency anaemia[12]
sarcoidosis
rickets
raised lead levels[12]
handicapping conditions
stress symptoms (adolescents)

USE OF THE NHS

More GP consultations than for the indigenous population, home visits less. In Bradford, Asians tend to consult only for physical symptoms and their hospital referrals are less than that of the indigenous population[13].

Asians and West Indians have low compliance and high defaulter rates. Both groups have a tendency to visit 'private' doctors. There is also a tendency to 'shop around' particularly with handicapped children, seeking a 'cure'.

Attendance of both groups for preventive care appears to relate to the attitudes and organization of family doctors, and their understanding of cultural patterns.

PRESENT AND FUTURE

Family doctors and the primary care team cannot cure or even help all the ills to which immigrant children under their care are subject. But they can try and understand their special problems and offer compassionate advice and help. There is a very special need to help parents to ensure that their children achieve their full potential. They are the citizens of tomorrow and need to be educated, trained and equipped to be happy and useful members of a multiracial society. 'The coloured family is accepted by medicine, as it ought to be by the whole of our society, as different, equal and deserving of the best'[14].

References

1. Mead, M. (1963). *Growing up in New Guinea.* (Harmondsworth, Middlesex: Pelican)
2. Lipton, E. L., Steinschneider, A. and Richmond, S. B. R. (1965). Swaddling, a child care practice: historical cultural experimental observations. *Paediatrics* (Suppl.), **35**, 521
3. De Mause, L. (ed.) (1974). History of Childhood (London: Condor Books, Souvenir Press (E & A Ltd.)
4. Vernon, P. E. (1969). *Intelligence and Cultural Environment.* (London: Methuen)
5. Pollak, M. (1979). *Nine Years Old.* (Lancaster: MTP Press)
6. Rutter, M. *et al.* (1974). Children of West Indian immigrants. I. Rates of behavioural deviance and psychological disorder. *J. Child. Psychol. Psychiatr.*, **15**, 241
7. Rutter, M. and Madge, N. (1976). *Cycles of Disadvantage.* (London: Heinemann)
8. *Social Trends 15* (1985). (London: HMSO)
9. Yule, W. *et al.* (1975). Children of West Indian immigrants. 2. Intellectual performance and reading attainment. *J. Child Psychol. Psychiatr.*, **16**, 1
10. Townsend, H. E. R. (1971). *Immigrant Pupils in England The L.E.A. Response.* (Slough: NFER)
11. Lord Scarman (1981). *The Brixton Disorders.* (London: HMSO)
12. Lobo, E. de H. (1978). *Children of Immigrants to Britain: their Health and Social Problems.* (London: Hodder & Stoughton)
13. Rack, P. (1978). Immigrant Children and the Health Service. Report of the *68th Annual Conference of the National Association for Maternal and Child Welfare*
14. Editorial (1973). *Gen. Practit.*, Feb. 16th

28

Housing

It may seem a truism that 'there is no place like home' but, in fact, the effect which housing has upon families, their lives, well-being and health is extremely complex. Many research papers have associated 'poor' housing with such varied factors as:

perinatal mortality
child abuse
degree of handicap
poor speech
poor reading skills
health and growth of the mother
bad temper
delinquency
accidents
psychiatric illness

Yet the exact features of poor housing which produced these effects are far from clear. So many of these conditions are also closely associated with low income and social class and the effect which housing, as such, exerts is difficult to elucidate.

Poor housing, poor amenities and poor neighbourhood are most commonly associated with:

low income families
low social class
fatherless families
immigrant families (Figure 28.1)

Homelessness is associated with:

fatherless families
families with young children
large families

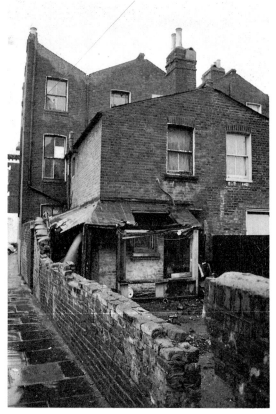

Figure 28.1 Multi-occupied slum dwelling, all families immigrants.

SOME EFFECTS OF HOUSING WHICH ARE CLEARLY ESTABLISHED

Rehousing

Usually a short period of sadness, even mourning, for the lost surroundings is quickly replaced by adaptation to the new; the outcome is satisfaction with the new housing and often better schools for the children.

It is the layout of the surroundings and social composition of the new neighbourhood that are more important than the structure of the house.

Sometimes, rehousing is associated with higher rents and one consequence may be fathers working longer hours and being less at home.

Their wives are thus more alone and when this is accompanied by poor transport to shops which are further away than the 'corner' shop and perhaps there is a greater distance to travel to parents, the isolation may lead to depression.

Design of house and estate

Studies[1, 2] from America have equated large, unimaginative housing estates, although with good amenities, with feelings of impersonalization, high levels of vandalism and delinquency.

Hammersmith Borough showed that people who were rehoused to small housing estates with easy access to other neighbourhoods were more satisfied with their lives, had more social life and friends than those rehoused on to larger housing estates[3].

Many writers have stressed the need for privacy and a 'defensive space'. It would appear that this is one of the definite factors in housing which affects the occupiers. It is the *personal* overcrowding which is more important than the *density* of people in the area, e.g. although flat dwellers suffer more noise disturbance than house dwellers, it is not the noise they complain about, but the fact that they themselves cannot make noise[4, 5].

Poor design causing accidents to children in the home has already been mentioned.

Pollak's study[6] of 173 Brixton children found only 18% of the 9-year-old West Indian children, compared with 87% of English 9-year-olds, had a toy cupboard or special place to keep their toys and belongings. No place to call your own is hardly conducive to learning a sense of, or respect for, property.

The Townsend study showed 44% of social class 4 and 5 had no safe place in which to live.

High-rise flats

Much of the evidence is conflicting. There is general agreement that the majority of mothers with preschool children dislike living above ground level; this dissatisfaction decreases as the children grow older. The incidence both of maternal depression and psychoneurosis is higher in mothers living in flats compared with those who live in houses.

Overcrowding

It is not difficult to imagine, where overcrowding exists, that different people have to undertake different activities, in the small crowded space (Figure 28.2). This is likely to result in bad and frayed tempers

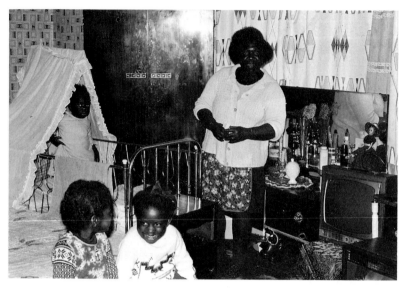

Figure 28.2   Two parents and three children live in this one room.

in parents and in children. The children will become restless. Older children will want to get out of the home. Parents can exert less control.

It is not surprising that the following are associated with overcrowding:

poor language development
poor educational progress
psychiatric disturbance in parent and child
frequent URTI, especially in the first year of life.

Housing and the poverty trap

Families on low income find that although they may cut down on food and clothes, rent cannot be reduced. The poorer the family, the higher the proportion of the income is taken up by rent.

Families on low income will find it impossible to obtain mortgages.

Thus poor families cannot buy their houses and, in addition, keep the property in good repair.

The majority of families who live in furnished accommodation are poor and deprived, yet furnished rooms carry a higher rent, proportionately, compared with unfurnished.

SPECIAL EFFECTS

It is established that overcrowded, inadequate housing is associated with poor educational achievement and delinquency in children but current evidence suggests that mothers are even more adversely affected by their housing conditions than their children. This is, perhaps, not surprising. Women are probably especially susceptible to a lack of 'defensive space'. It may affect their general well-being. We know that they are likely to suffer depression and psychosomatic illnesses when housing conditions are poor. Furthermore, if their housing is poor, they are more likely to be single parents – a stress factor in itself. What is not yet researched is what effect a depressed or psychologically disturbed mother has upon her children.

Pollak studied the development of four different groups of 3-year-olds, living in town, country, England and USA. Their developmental levels were not related to the adequacy or inadequacy of their housing, and their development was little affected by housing conditions[7].

Developmental scales matched against the housing and maternal care scales[7]

	English	West Indian	American	
			White	Negro
Housing				
Motor	NS	NS	NS	NS
Personal-social	NS	NS	NS	NS
Language	NS	$p < 0.05$	NS	NS
Adaptive	NS	NS	NS	NS
Maternal care				
Motor	NS	$p < 0.05$	NS	NS
Personal-social	$p < 0.01$	$p < 0.001$	$p < 0.001$	$p < 0.001$
Language	$p < 0.001$	$p < 0.001$	$p < 0.001$	$p < 0.001$
Adaptive	$p < 0.01$	$p < 0.001$	$p < 0.001$	$p < 0.001$

However, when developmental achievements of the same four groups were matched against the levels of their maternal care, their development was highly significantly related. The study showed that the adage, 'There is no place like home', is only likely to be true when it contains an adequate mother.

References

1. Yancey, W. L. (1976). Architecture: interaction and social control. In Kalt and Zalkind (eds.) *Urban Problems*. (New York: Oxford University Press)
2. Hartman, C. W. (1976). Social values and housing orientations. In Kalt and Zalkind (eds.) *Urban Problems*. (New York: Oxford University Press)
3. *Living in a Council Flat* (1974). (London Borough of Hammersmith)
4. Newman, D. (1976). Defensible space. In Kalt and Zalkind (eds.) *Urban Problems*. (New York: Oxford University Press)
5. Canter, D. (1974). Empirical research in environmental psychology. *Bull. Br. Psychol. Soc.*, **2**, 31
6. Pollak, M. (1979). *Nine Years Old*. (Lancaster: MTP Press)
7. Pollak, M. (1979). Housing and mothering. *Arch. Dis. Child.*, **54**, 54-58

SECTION V

Uses of . . .

Many patients and some doctors still have the belief that management of children's problems requires the doctors to take action and use a range of possibilities. Yet often the best care is through the use of inaction or seemingly to be 'doing nothing' – which requires considerable restraint and discipline by the doctor.

Nevertheless, most consultations involve 'doing something' and/or the use of some physical action or some agency, so it is useful to examine the best ways of making use of available choices.

In an Utopian purely scientific world diseases would be treated using necessary and proven measures and non-diseases would be left untreated but managed appropriately.

In our real-life situation it is the management of child and family that are the first priority with the disease assuming secondary importance.

An ability to see 'the wood for the trees' is needed in practice to see the needs of a particular child within the context of his family milieu. Even with potentially life-threatening conditions such as leukaemia, for example, sensitive and sensible human care is of prime importance.

29

Use of drugs

Even before prescribing anything at all the doctor should ask himself what is it for and what it is *not* for? If a placebo, is it for mum, dad, granny, doctor or the child? Is it safe?

WHEN TO PRESCRIBE?

Use of drugs fits into these groups:

curative drugs
symptomatic relieving drugs
placebos

Specific curative drugs are necessary when a specific condition known to require specific therapy has been diagnosed. In childhood the most likely indications for curative therapy are infections requiring antibiotics. However, it is by no means agreed that all infections demand antibiotics (see p. 111). Many infections will resolve satisfactorily without antibiotics such as common upper respiratory infections, minor skin infections and gastrointestinal infections.

Symptom-relieving drugs make up most of the prescribing for children. Decisions on whether they should or should not be prescribed is a decision for each doctor and each parent. Most disorders of children are self-resolving and will do so without drugs – the question to be asked is whether the weight of evidence against prescribing symptom relievers is so strong as to withhold relief? Probably pain must be relieved but what about symptoms such as cough, sickness, diarrhoea, not sleeping and not eating?

Comforters – placebos – there is a thin line between symptom-relieving drugs and placebos that are prescribed with known intention of pleasing the parent, child and/or doctor. Many symptom relievers are placebos and it can be argued that many placebos can act as symptom relievers.

There is a strong case for absolute honesty in medical practice. Therefore placebos must be dishonest and must never be prescribed. There is also a case put forward for prescribing of placebos that are harmless and can do no harm if they please and assist in promoting a satisfactory outcome.

It is argued also by the antiplacebo lobby that the custom of prescribing placebos will lead to over-dependence and over-demands by patients.

The debate over use of placebos has to be resolved individually but knowledgeably by each doctor. Their use is not bad practice providing that the decision to use them is made positively and in awareness that they are what they are.

It is noticeable that young doctors come to general practice strongly antiplacebo – yet with personal patient responsibilities they often change their views and join the placebo prescribers.

Not only is it extremely difficult for the doctor to prescribe nothing but it is often unacceptable for some parents, who find comfort for their own stresses in their child's medicine. Some parents are unable to manage their own everyday lives, let alone their child's sickness. They need the prop of some medicine for their sick child.

WHEN *NOT* TO PRESCRIBE?

As in all branches of medicine a diagnosis, however vague and inaccurate, must precede treatment so a prescription should only be given when a diagnosis has been made.

It is unwise and may be dangerous to prescribe for symptoms that may be the earliest features of an unsuspected major serious disease. For example, treating abdominal pain, vomiting and diarrhoea with a 'blind' prescription may lead to a life-threatening situation if an acute appendicitis is missed or not thought of. A knowledge of the child and family and past reactions to illness is particularly helpful.

It is much better practice to explain the situation to the mother and arrange for a reassessment within a short while.

WHAT TO PRESCRIBE FOR COMMON DISEASES OF CHILDREN?

Each doctor should create his/her personal formulary. The fewer preparations that it includes the better. It is more reasonable to become familiar with a few well tried favourites than to be continually changing and even worse to rush into prescribing the 'latest', but as yet unproven, drugs.

We do not propose to make out any list of personally recommended drugs because few others would agree with it. Rather we suggest that each one should consider the following categories and produce his/her own choices – not all will accept that each category requires any drugs. Beware of use of non-specifics in infants, i.e. analgesics, laxatives etc.

Pain relief

>   analgesic – decide on what is appropriate for different age groups (paracetamol is more favoured now than aspirin, but generally aspirin is safe and effective).

Anti-infective

>   antibiotics   ⎫ important to know the local common causal
>   chemotherapy ⎭ organisms and their sensitivities

Gastrointestinal

>   gastric sedative
>   antidiarrhoea
>   laxative (tablet, medicine or suppository?)
>   antispasmodic

Cough, cold, catarrh, sore throat

>   cough medicine
>   antispasmodic
>   nasal drops
>   lozenge, pastille

Wheezy chests

> antispasmodics
> inhalant drugs

Allergy

> antihistamines
> others

Fever

> antipyretic

Skin

Applications for:

> eczema
> nappy rash
> warts

Eye

> for conjunctivitis

Not sleeping

> hypnotic or sedative?

'Tonic'

> what if any? Should one accede to some parent's wishes?

Practical measures

Whenever a medicine is prescribed remember to:

> explain why it is given and with what expectations

> instruct how and how much to give and when – how to use spoonfuls, nasal drops, suppositories and skin preparations

mention possible side-effects

assess benefits or non-benefits of the preparations that are pre-scribed

enquire on compliance (many mums do not give their child the medicine prescribed)

consider proper dosages, particularly in first 6 months of life

How often on home visits does one see an array of past treatments on the mantelpiece? It has even been known for doctors to take the paediatric antibiotic languishing in the 'fridge for their own sore throat!

30

Use of 'the team'

The doctor cannot provide good care working alone. He needs to collaborate with others at the primary and other levels of care. Within most practices there are others involved:

receptionists
health visitors
nurses
social workers
occasionally, physiotherapists

However, the most important member of the team who is not usually listed is the *mother*, who must be considered as a team member.

Each member has his/her roles and parts to play.

Receptionist

She is the true person of first contact in the practice. As well as making appointments etc. she is the source of much advice, support and guidance.

Ideally, she is a cool, calm and caring mature person who has to deal skilfully with all human weaknesses, as well as strengths. She has to learn to be firm but helpful. The receptionist is the real shop front of the practice. She is very important and 'sans pareil' when good.

Over the years mothers and receptionists get to know one another well and she can become an 'auntie' to generations of mothers and children. Beware of giving the receptionist too much and unfair responsibilities. She is not a doctor or a nurse and thus it is wrong to expect her to give advice with the doctor's support. It is the doctor who is ultimately responsible for his receptionists' actions.

Health visitor

She is attached to a practice and is a key member of the team. She is involved with providing support and advice to the mother from the antenatal period onwards. The antenatal clinic allows her to get to know the mother *before* the birth of the baby and to discuss child-rearing practices, feeding problems and how family roles can expect to change with the arrival of a new baby, such as the effects on siblings. Future family size and spacing can also be discussed when the mother is particularly susceptible to guidance.

She has the statutory responsibilities to visit each new baby at home and keep in contact thereafter. She is able to dispense much sound commonsense advice on feeding and health in general. She should be actively involved in the child care arrangements of the practice, holding her own 'clinics' and meeting the doctors, receptionists, nurses and social workers regularly.

In some authorities there are special health visitors for particular groups such as the handicapped, spastic and athetoid patients, helping with feeding advice, changing catheters, knowing how Spitz valves work, etc.

Nurse

The attached *'district nurse'* has little to do with the care of healthy normal children but deals often with children who are chronically ill at home, providing care by visiting when required.

It is a source of aggravation that although nurses in hospital give injections all the time, many Health Authorities do not allow 'practice attached' nurses to give immunization injections.

The *'practice nurse'* employed by the practice is more involved with work in the practice premises than in the community. Like the receptionist she gets to know mothers and children well through her contacts at the practice child health clinics where she often administers immunizations. She becomes a well-known and respected figure in the practice. However, the limitations of the nurse's roles and work have to be accepted and she should not be put in situations which are more appropriate and correct for the doctor to handle.

Social workers

They have chosen to remain remote from family practice work. Their involvement usually begins only when social problems occur within the families. This is a great pity because they could contribute much in collaboration with the primary care team for disadvantaged families. Their involvement in child abuse and in placing children into care is usually remote from the general practices. These and other problem families are all patients of the practices and close co-operation between mutually respected professions would be of great benefit to all.

In the few practices where social workers are recognized members of 'the team', better care and services are provided with much saving of time and resources.

Doctors

The doctors are members of the team and not necessarily the unelected supremos. True team work has to be 'worked' for, because then the team functions best.

31

Use of the hospital

The hospital provides secondary care. It is at the district general hospital where the general specialist services are based, including paediatrics. Teaching hospitals provide super-specialist and regional facilities.

Although relatively few children are referred to hospital each year by the general practitioner, close inter-relationships are essential for good care. Gulfs and barriers still exist, however, and in the future a more integrated system of child care involving specialists more in the community and general practitioners in the hospital would seem appropriate.

The general practitioner cherishes a tried and trusted paediatrician whom he can turn to for advice and support and who will be willing to visit at home on the rare occasions when this is necessary.

WHY TO REFER TO HOSPITAL AND WHEN?

Before referring any patient to hospital it may be good discipline to ask oneself – why?

Is it for expert knowledge?
Is it for an investigation not possible in practice?
Is it because the patient cannot be treated at home?
Is it because the patient's anxiety has not been allayed?
Is this a normal family with an abnormal problem or an abnormal family with a normal problem?

OR

Is it for more egotistic reasons not directly related to patient care and help?

The chief reasons for the general practitioner referring a child to a hospital specialist are when the child's condition needs hospital care and/or investigations are necessary. The decision as to *when* is left to the individual practitioner. There is a wide range in the referral rates between general practitioners depending on many personal factors, such as age and length of qualification and paediatric experience.

In addition to referral when advice and care are required to investigate and treat special conditions, hospital admission may be necessary on social grounds, when some parents find it difficult to cope with an illness that others might manage well at home. It is important for hospital (especially junior) staff to appreciate this. Referral is sometimes important as a therapeutic measure in itself. The 'therapeutic referral' is helpful when the situation is such that the practitioner knows the diagnosis and has applied the appropriate management, but the mother, father or grandparents need second opinion reassurance from a 'specialist'. Such referrals must not be considered failures by the practitioner – rather the doctor becomes sensitive to the family's need, even pre-empting the parents' request. For example, take note when father comes too! The reasons for referral to, and the actions expected from, the consultant need stating in the referral letter. (Always assume that the letter may be opened and read by parents!)

Referrals to hospital need to be explained to parents. Such is the selling power of hospital medicine, that referral is tantamount to cure in the minds of some – including paramedicals. A discussion of what the hospital and specialist has to offer, what investigations might be undertaken, what outcome is expected etc., is needed so that parents have realistic expectations of the hospital referral.

Examples are:

Chronic asthma, when parents seek frequent re-referrals because of persistent attacks and have not yet accepted the chronic nature of the disease.

Handicapped children: their parents often 'shop around' looking for a cure.

Mentally retarded children. In over 90% of mental retardation no cause can be found, but it is very understandable for parents to wish every investigative stone to be turned or second or third opinions sought before accepting the diagnosis. Such parents need constant reassurance and explanation; they need to be reassured that it is 'not their fault'. The paediatrician and family doctor must liaise to support the family.

WHAT TO REFER?

There are at least four types of problems that need referral.

Emergencies

These may be medical, surgical or social. The welfare and safety of the child are of prime importance, and if the doctor believes that a potentially serious and dangerous condition *may* be present then it is safer and better to admit the child for observation, even if later in retrospect such admission may not have been necessary.

'GP stuck'

This is when the practitioner requires specialist experience and expertise to elucidate the matter.

Domiciliary consultation

The domiciliary consultation offers the opportunity for paediatrician and family doctor to meet at the home and to meet parents for discussion and explanation. It is also, now, a rarity.

Technological procedure

Often referral to a specialist is necessary for confirmatory investigations or surgical procedures requiring special expertise not possible in the primary care setting.

Therapeutic referral

See p. 232.

TO WHOM?

An important skill of the general practitioner is to know the pros and cons of specialists at the local district general hospital or in other units, and to discover from experience who knows what and does things best and to learn of the specialists' views and likely procedures. Thus, not all ENT surgeons deal with glue ears in the same ways, nor do all ophthalmologists manage squints identically, nor do all psychiatrists approach school refusals alike.

The child's problem may require certain special skills possessed by a particular specialist.

The specialist's and the parents' personalities may require careful matching.

Other factors in the choice will be the services that the local hospital provide – such as waiting time, communication, in-patient facilities and follow-up arrangements.

Communications should be through personal contacts or through personal letters, typed or handwritten, rather than by pre-printed multiple choice question forms provided by the hospital and audited by a hospital booking clerk.

It has to be accepted that in many districts there is no real choice because of the small number of specialists available.

WHAT TO SAY?

Good communications between the various parties – practitioner, specialist and parents – are *sine qua non*.

The mother must be kept informed and clear explanations given at all stages.

The general practitioner in his referral letter (or telephone call) should state clearly why the referral is being made, provide information on the social and family background and express his (GP's) expectations from the referral.

Provided that mutual relations are good between specialist and practitioner then it is in order for the latter to 'instruct' his specialist colleague on what is expected from the consultation.

The paediatrician must communicate his findings and opinion quickly, and send a final discharge letter.

USE OF PATHOLOGY DEPARTMENT

Many investigations are unpleasant and frightening to the child especially when needles are used. Therefore the benefits from the investigations must be tempered by convincing expectation from the tests. A history and examination are usually sufficient in management of common paediatric conditions and investigations should be used with discrimination and not as routine batteries. The most frequent tests are urinalysis, haemoglobin and other haematological tests; less frequently biochemical tests. Obviously, the laboratory is used more in cases being treated at home.

USE OF RADIOLOGICAL DEPARTMENT

Though less unpleasant because painful procedures are not often necessary, nevertheless, the experience may be frightening for the child. Therefore pause before referring to ensure that the procedure is really necessary.

X-rays to check for possible bone fractures are the most frequent; chest radiography may be of value to check on possible persisting lung infections, but contrast media radiography is only rarely necessary direct from general practice.

Much has been written of the necessity of full investigations of every urinary infection. This necessity is probably overrated.

32

Use of practice clinics

For effective and efficient child care involving the most economic use of resources, practice clinics are recommended for all but the smallest practices (Figure 32.1).

The practice clinic brings together the members of the health team as well as parents and children. It provides opportunities for concentration of interests as well as resources.

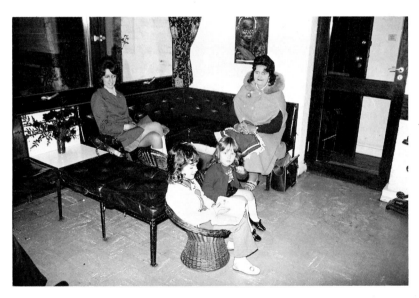

Figure 32.1

ANTENATAL CLINIC

It is during the antenatal period that mothers are receptive to learning and influence. An important member of the practice antenatal clinic is the *health visitor* who is able to get to know her future mothers and they her. Mothers see the same doctor, midwife, health visitor and receptionists.

At each attendance the opportunities should be taken to reassure and encourage the mother and to discuss with her baby feeding and rearing practices, the effects of a new baby on the family and family size and planning.

WELL CHILD CLINIC

A definite practice routine should be in force. Mothers should be encouraged to attend as soon as they are ambulant following delivery, from 2 to 4 weeks, for general assessment from and discussion with the practitioner and/or health visitor. Arrangements for regular attendance are necessary and follow-up reminders are needed for defaulters.

There should be opportunities for:

discussing feeding problems

asking how mum and baby are getting along

giving mum a forum for airing problems, physical and psychological, relating to both the baby and herself, asking about physical and psychological problems

measuring baby's height, weight and head circumference

surveillance of development at regular times

immunizations

DEVELOPMENTAL SURVEILLANCE

This is probably best done by doctors and health visitors who have the training and time.

IMMUNIZATION CLINICS

These can be combined with well-child sessions or organized separately by the practice nurse – but there should always be a doctor available when such a clinic is in progress.

MOTHERS' GROUPS

Chapman[1] reports improved mother/child relationships, less surgery attendances for psychological problems and, perhaps most important, friendships arising between the visiting mothers.

When social workers are attached to primary care teams in greater numbers, it would seem that this must be one of their first priorities.

Reference

1. Chapman, B. (1984). Mother and baby groups in general practice. In Gray, D. P. (ed.) *The Medical Annual.* (Bristol: Wright)

33

Use of surveillance

DEVELOPMENTAL SURVEILLANCE

Clinical medicine depends on adding up symptoms and signs to make a diagnosis.

In paediatrics, a developmental diagnosis is made by matching the stage of development of a particular child against what is known to be 'average' for the child's age. Thus measurement in one of the parameters of development will give a measure of achievement in that area. A differential diagnosis can be made by assessing levels of development in all parameters of development and comparing these with each other.

Developmental surveillance should be seen as measuring levels of achievements in developmental parameters.

Developmental assessment is a specialized, in-depth, measurement of developmental parameters, together with testing other factors which may have affected development such as neurological function and maturity, genetic, familial and environmental factors, and sensory intactness.

SURVEILLANCE IN THE COMMUNITY

Test for Common Problems

Severe deafness is likely to be encountered only every 15 years in an average-sized practice. Otitis media, on the other hand, is likely to leave residual deafness in approximately 17% of cases. It is much more worthwhile to test for the latter than the former.

Test from Birth to School Age

Several studies from general practice[1-3] have shown that the highest returns in abnormalities occur not only in the first year of life but also between 3 and 5 years. It is therefore more effective to offer surveillance to older ages.

The lovely baby in Figure 33.1 has no perinatal risk factors, no environmental risk factors, yet he is *at risk* of developing myopia at a later age *because* both his parents are wearing glasses. A family picture like this should alert the doctor to screening this child's visual acuity from 3 years onwards.

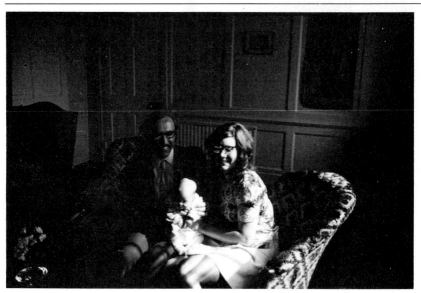

Figure 33.1

Look at factors other than classical developmental examinations in the clinic

When the children are developing well, reassurance of the parents is a most important part of the clinic. Anything which enhances parents' confidence in their parenting skills is worthwhile.

Cheryl has a spastic quadriplegia. She is one of the lucky 40% of cases with a normal IQ. It is important to help her parents to provide stimulation for her normal IQ but taking her physical problems into account.

Parent counselling is another part of the surveillance clinic.

J.P. (Figure 33.2) has an abnormality of his megakaryocytes and absence of his radii. He is also mentally retarded. It is helpful to counsel his mother at each visit to prepare her acceptance for J.P.'s attendance at a special school.

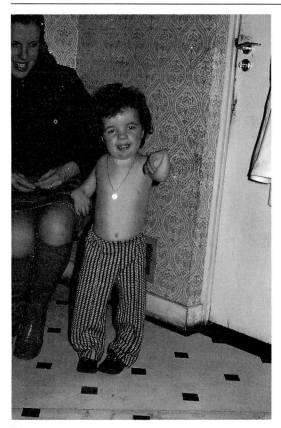

Figure 33.2

Common needs of the handicapped

Due to the small numbers of each handicap which generalists are likely to encounter, they cannot become specialists in each handicap. However, all handicapped children have some common needs and surveillance clinics in the community can help to provide these. For example:

One handicap is more likely to be associated with another, therefore needs searching for.

Paul (Figure 33.3) has a hemiplegia and shows a well-known associated handicap – a strabismus.

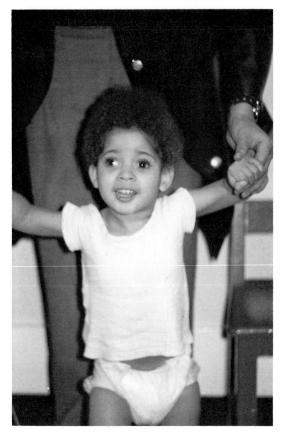

Figure 33.3

Although often late, handicapped children *do* pass their milestones and by drawing attention to this, parental encouragement ensues.

WHO SHOULD DO IT?

Does it really matter as long as it is well done? There are advantages if:

The same person sees the child each time to maintain continuity and assess progress.

This is someone who knows not only the baby but also the family.

The surveillance is part of a comprehensive, preventive service, i.e. in general practice the same doctor might have conducted some of the antenatal examinations as well.

The ideal is if there can be prevention, diagnosis and treatment available in the same clinic.

The same doctor can see the child in health and in sickness.

SURVEILLANCE FOR WHOM?

There is no question that surveillance should be available for 100% of the children of the practice.

It is a matter of concern that so often it is the defaulters who are the children who most need to be seen. There is a need for some register to be kept of the population at risk, matched against those who came and that the clinic has a policy towards these defaulters.

Several workers[2] have shown it is possible to achieve high attendance rates even in 'inner city' areas, but this is not achieved without much effort and personal 'persuasion'.

WHAT TO DO?

Growth and motor skills

Height, weight, head circumference (see pages 25, 36, 40, 41)
Gross motor
    locomotion
    balance
Fine motor
    hand and finger function

Personal and social skills

Personal
    development of personality
    development of independence
    relationship with parents and siblings
    eating, sleeping
    sphincter control

Social
  recognition of others
  play and behaviour to others
  acceptance of social and cultural mores

Language development

comprehension
expression
symbolic (see page 62)

Non-verbal skills

non-verbal problem-solving with bricks, shapes and drawing

WHEN TO REFER?

There will be variation in the referral of developmental problems according to the experience, skills and inclination of the doctor, but the following is a sensible list for definite referral:

3 months

Cannot raise head when in prone.
Does not appear to listen to mother's voice or react to loud noises.
Does not focus on mother's eyes.

6 months

Cannot arch back and extend arms when prone with head up.
Cannot sit, although may need back support.
Does not smile or laugh.
Is not babbling.
Never reaches out for a toy.
Never turns to mother's voice.
Is not visually alert.
Has a squint and/or nystagmus.

1 year

Cannot pull to stand.
Cannot pick up Smarties with finger and thumb apposition.
Cannot follow a small rolling ball at a distance and does not fixate onto small objects.
Squint.
Is not making distinguishable sounds or words.
Does not turn quickly and accurately to the human voice.
Shows no interest in play objects.

18 months

Is not walking around furniture.
Is not mobile on the floor.
No finger thumb apposition.
Not beginning to feed self.
Cannot fixate on and pick up hundreds and thousands, or squint.
Has no single word, is not using jargon.
Cannot accurately locate whisper.

2 years

Cannot get on and off a chair.
Cannot unscrew easy bottle top.
Goes up close to the television.
Is not putting two words together and does not appear to hear soft sounds.
Is not interested in toys, particularly simple shape matching.

3 years

Cannot undress fully and dress except buttons and zips.
Cannot stand on one leg.
Is not making sentences of three words.
Has echolalia.
Is not interested in other children and outsiders.
Has repetitive or rocking movements.
Cannot play meaningfully with constructive toys.

4 years

Flits from one thing to another.

'On the go' all day.

Speech is bizarre.

History of otitis media, appears deaf and has poor language development.

Has less than 6/9 vision in either eye and 9 for near vision.

Does not play imaginative games with other children and is anti-social.

References

1. Curtis Jenkins, G. (1977). Surveillance of pre-school children in general practice. In Drullien and Drummond (eds.) *Neurodevelopmental Problems in Early Childhood.* (Oxford: Blackwell)
2. Pollak, M. (1984). Family practice and development. In *The Medical Annual.* (Bristol: Wright)
3. Hooper, P. (1977). Developmental screening. In Hart, C. (ed.) *Child Care in General Practice.* (Edinburgh: Churchill Livingstone)

34

Use of community clinics

In an ideal state there should be no need for general community children's clinics. All general child case services should be carried out from general practice.

However, in health care systems where practitioners are free to arrange and organize their work as they desire and mothers are to be free to choose the services for their children, there is no total cover from general practice.

In order that child care services be available for mothers and children whose practitioners have no such services community child health clinics have to be provided.

These duplicate the work of other practices in the district but this is inevitable.

Even where there are complete general child care services provided by general practitioners, there is need for specialist child development clinics to assess and manage particular problems of children – such as slow development, major handicaps and learning and social problems.

SECTION VI

The Whole Child

35

The whole child

Good child care involves much more than prescribing for symptoms because common 'presenting symptoms' may be manifestations of hidden and deeper problems affecting not only the child but the whole family and their social environment.

Besides considering the clinical situation, further questions should be asked:

Why is the child being brought *now* and for *these* symptoms?

What is the demeanour and personality of the child and the mother (father)?

What does one know of past illnesses and symptoms?

What sort of family and under what conditions do they live?

(The last question illustrates the importance of using home visits by doctor and/or health visitor to learn about home circumstances.)

It is important, then, to understand:

the *child* as a whole person

the *family* as a unit but to include extensions – grandparents, uncles, aunts and cousins.

the *social circumstances* in which they live and the opportunities offered for the child to develop individually.

WHAT ARE THE AIMS OF CHILD CARE?

The *child* should be happy and healthy. This depends on sound and commonsense parenthood but also on close collaboration with professional services.

Together parents and professionals must emphasize:

preventive measures

checks on normal development
appropriate management of common disorder
appreciation of normal abnormalities and understanding of the natural patterns and history of child development and disorders

The *family* has to accept its roles and responsibilities for self-care and self-help.

Social care involves the 'art of the possible' and making the best use of available local and family resources – which will always be less than optimal.

The *objectives of child care* can be summarized as:

physical care and protection
affection, love and approval
stimulation and teaching
standards of behaviour, discipline and control
encouragement of self-confidence and autonomy

WHO IS INVOLVED?

Levels of care, each with their own roles and responsibilities, must be recognized.

Self-care – within the family unit is the basic first level of care and its quality and effectiveness depend on the capability, skills and knowledge of the parents and others in the extended family. Time and attention should be spent on teaching future and present families on elements of *good* sound child care and what can and should be done by whom, when, where and how.

Primary professional care is that care to which parents have direct access and who provide first contact and often long term continuing care.

There are many possible sources:

general practitioners
health visitors
social workers/services
community clinics
hospital accident–emergency departments
school health services

These have their own contents and limitations of care, which in an ideal setting should work closely and harmoniously – but they rarely do so.

SECONDARY SPECIALIST SERVICES

Such services are based on large populations, such as those of a district general hospital or social service department, and children with special problems are referred to them from the primary care level.

Their roles are to sort out and deal with particular problems and then to refer the child and family back to the primary care professionals. Except in particular circumstances, such as some chronic disorders, the specialist units do not undertake long term continuing care.

IS THERE A NEED FOR A GENERALIST?

In the age of ever-increasing specialism, is there a need for a generalist paediatrician?

Why do generalists never win Nobel prizes?

Is it possible to practise both high technology and holistic paediatrics?

Advantages of a Generalist

Generalists are particularly important in the case of children who are growing and developing and therefore have changing needs; more so in the case of handicap, when several or many different body systems are involved as well as differing needs at different developmental levels.

A generalist sees it as his/her remit to see the whole family and the whole child. The medical history and psychological make-up of several members of the family are probably well known.

We have already emphasized the importance of family, environment and social factors on health. They are equally important in illness. A generalist expects to take all these factors into account.

It is an advantage to a patient to be treated as an individual whose background is either already known or is studied, suffering a disease process. It is difficult for high technology specialists with vast knowledge of certain types of disease to look at the problem this way.

The generalist, holistic paediatrician learns to treat some symptoms and signs as *only* symptoms and to look beyond for a diagnosis. Examples are: anaemia, speech delay, failure to thrive.

However, the holistic paediatrician is only at best when he/she is offering continuity of care. This certainly is what the patient needs, someone who knows their past, their present and who will be available in the future. This ideal is never realized, but holistic doctors must have it as an aim.

The generalist must know when, to whom and why to refer to the specialist. We have already discussed referral to hospital (pp. 233–4) and emphasize it is part of the generalist's job to know available consultants and their work.

At present, the majority of psychosocial problems are dealt with by the generalist. There may be a case for expert advice, particularly in behavioural problems[1] being used more often than at present – or generalists learning more treatment methods.

THE DOCTOR AS THE LEADER OF THE TEAM?

Is a leader needed? Many would deny this. We do not agree. Someone has to lead a group, that is the leader.

Groups and teams want a leader. The buck has to stop somewhere. Leaders often need to set an example, especially to young inexperienced members of the team, in caring and attitudes towards social class 5 patients, aggressive patients, alcoholics, the old and poor.

Who in the primary care team has responsibility for patients 24 hours per day and 365 days per year? How can team decisions be made in the middle of a night visit?

There is an obvious need for all members of the primary care team to agree on some common policies, so that similar advice on subjects such as infant feeding, nocturnal enuresis, etc. is given by each member of the team.

SHOULD THE WHOLE PAEDIATRICIAN INFLUENCE HIS PATIENTS AND PARENTS, AND HOW?

Purists may take the view that doctors should confine themselves to the management of illness. We believe otherwise.

It is desirable for the holistic paediatrician to give advice not only on feeding and health problems, but also on child-rearing methods, the importance of learning to learn, etc. It is unrealistic to expect that every woman who delivers of a baby automatically both wishes and knows how to provide the loving stimulating environment which her baby needs.

The paediatrician must guard against giving advice which is loaded with his/her own views, rather giving sound data based on proven ideas. He will remember that because children are developing they are more susceptible to influence than when mature.

Paediatricians have added responsibilities due to the youth of their patients. They need to ask themselves:

Is parental consent always required?

Should one ever examine, assess or immunize without both the presence and consent of the parent? Is the doctor ever *in locus parentis?*

Does the doctor believe in positive discrimination? Is there a case to be made for extra help in social disprivilege or do all children have to be treated exactly the same?

WHERE TO CARE?

Whatever the details of a local system of child care it is most important that parents should know their way around the services and to be familiar with ways in which to obtain access to care. This may be to know how to get to the general practice, to the local clinic (if used), to the social services department and to the local hospital accident-emergency department. It is up to the professionals to inform parents of local arrangements, preferably by some written instructions which can be kept for reference.

WHAT PROBLEMS?

The common clinical problems have been noted but there may be hidden occult factors, therefore characteristic leading signals should be noted and followed up.

Why has the child been brought now with this particular problem?

Why is mother such a frequent attender for apparent 'minor' conditions?

Why has father come too?

Why has child been brought by sibling, father, grandmother or child-minder?

Why these particular behavioural symptoms (if present)?

What is the nature of the situation and condition?

What should be done now and later?

HOW TO CARE?

To make best use of the many and varied resources, attention must be paid to coordination and collaboration between them but also that each professional service resource should have its own policies, plans and targets for care.

Each practice, each specialist unit and each district should have recognized and agreed policies for:

neonatal care
infant care
pre-school care
school care
adolescent care
care of handicapped and chronically ill children

– as well as for defined conditions and syndromes such as ear disorders and deafness, asthma, eczema, enuresis, non-thriving, epilepsy and convulsions.

CHRONIC ILLNESS NEEDS A PLAN

Unless continuing care ensues, an initial assessment is almost worthless.

Many health districts have assessment centres for handicapped and developmentally delayed children. Unless these are combined with treatment and follow-up, assessment is a sterile exercise. Doctors may feel very proud to make the diagnosis of some rare, long-sounding syndrome. This is not what parents want. They want to know the prognosis and what is to be done.

Very often what they want and need is a small slice of the doctor's time – just to listen how unbearable it was that Johnny had yet another uncontrolled fit whilst she was alone in the house or how she hates all the neighbours knowing. Betty goes to school by school bus so they all know 'She's not normal'.

Regular follow-up helps to establish a trusting patient–doctor relationship.

Although the doctor is thinking ahead, it is best to keep the conversation mostly on present strengths, weaknesses and problems.

Help parents and child to have as normal a social life as is possible.

Always encourage the parents in their own parenting skills.

The aim is to end up as a friend to both child and parents as well as being their doctor.

WHY CARE – ITS QUALITY?

Provision of care is not sufficient. Its standards and quality must be measured and assessed wherever possible to allow providers to self-check their own profiles with those of others.

Measurement demands meaningful and reliable data and facts and these have to be collected and analysed. Indices of quality must be provided in non-threatening ways to encourage self-improvements and not as diktat directives.

Examples of indices on which data could be provided by NHS now are:

infant and child mortality rates
immunization rates
prescribing rates and content
hospital attendance/admission
local (district) rates of congenital dislocation of hip, undescended testes, non-accidental injuries
measles and whooping cough notification

Although the hard scientific medical approach to child care is accepted, the art of medicine includes the important techniques of communication, understanding and caring.

DO WE KNOW WHAT THE PATIENTS WANT?

Certainly they want care. They want a doctor who will treat them as individuals in the bosom of their own family surroundings. Their doctor must have a wide knowledge and be a wise counsellor.

CHILDREN'S HERITAGE

Do we give priority to children's services, or do we only pay lip service? Children were a priority group until 1977, not so now.

Do children nowadays count for less, as Professor Meadows points out?[2] Until the last NHS reshuffle, children in each NHS health district had both a Specialist in Community Health (Child Health) and Area Nurse (Child Health). Until the Seebohm Report, social services had children's departments until the generic social worker came into being.

At the present time, the teachers, frustrated and angry, organize strikes which mean their pupils must lose precious schooling.

The Education Act has theoretically made provision for children with special needs but government has not provided the wherewithal to implement the plans.

Previous chapters have related the many ills and scourges to which children of today are 'at risk'. A disenchanted, disillusioned group of young people are growing up in our inner cities untrained and unfit to obtain worthwhile job opportunities and the first step on the ladder.

Something must be done. There are no miracles round the corner. Each and every one of us who works with children must do all we can to ensure that the nation's heritage grows up healthy, happy and able to fulfil its potential.

If we look at the frequency of one-parent families and divorce, we must realize that many children in the future will spend much of their lives growing up without one of their natural parents and, since re-marriage is common, with a step-parent and probably step-siblings.

Both mothers and fathers are getting younger, and are more likely to live away from grandparents and parents. They are likely to be inexperienced in life, let alone in child rearing.

Looking after children in the future one must realize that Britain today, as in many other developed countries, has gone a long way away from the happy unit family of mother, father, son and daughter. We must ensure that the needs of children are met.

Old words still ring true:

> 'To prevent whenever possible
> To cure sometimes
> To relieve often
> and
> To comfort always'

References

1. Graham, P. and Jenkins, S. (1985). *Arch. Dis. Child.*, **60**, 777
2. Meadows, J. (1985). And children first? *Arch. Dis. Child.*, **60**, 781–782

Appendix

Helping your child to talk – Advice to parents

Babies and small children learn to talk through contact with grown-ups. Moreover, they learn most from those persons who are closest to them. Naturally, these are usually their parents. All parents, therefore, have a very important role to play in their children's speech and language development. *You are your child's best teacher.*

There are a great many ways in which you can help. Here are some of them:

If you were prescribed medicine for your child, you would not hesitate to give it. Medicine does not help a child to talk, so the prescription is that you set aside 15 minutes of each day for 'talking' to your child. The physical contact is important, so sit with him on your knee. For small children, and those not yet talking, it is best to have a book with only one picture on a page. (The Ladybird books, which are available at many local stores, and are very inexpensive, are ideal.) Look carefully at each page, say the word, repeat it, and perhaps make some comment about it. For example 'Oh, look, the shoe is red'. Then repeat the word again. Turn over the page, and say the word of the next picture. Even if your child is not yet talking, there is no reason why this 'talking' medicine should not help. Do not try to make the child repeat the word, he will do so as soon as he is able. If he repeats the word but indistinctly, do not correct him, but repeat the word yourself, correctly pronounced.

For older children, a storybook is helpful. Read the same story every day, and, if possible, in the same way. Children love to hear the same story over and over again. When he has learned the story 'by heart' begin to ask him to fill in some words. 'Jack and Jill went up the ...' If he says the word, always repeat it after him – 'Yes, Jack and Jill went up the *hill*'.

When he has learned the nouns, begin on adverbs and adjectives. 'Jack and Jill went ... the hill'. 'Yes, Jack and Jill went *up* the hill'.

When you are very successful, your child will have taken over most of the story telling.

Try to get into the habit of having 'chatting' sessions. When you come in from an expedition, 'chat' about what you have seen and done. Shopping is another good time in which to 'chat' about the goods in the shops.

When you are doing your household work, you can try to make a talking game out of the jobs. Most little children love to help around the house, and you can make a routine of talking. 'First we turn the water on, not too hot and not too cold. Here comes the soap liquid, and here's the mop. It goes swish, swish around the cup. Now it's clean and you can wipe it dry.'

Let your child hear music and nursery rhymes. Even better, let him have a tape recorder of his own so that he can put on music for himself. Encourage him to sing and repeat rhymes whenever you can. It is very helpful to include some physical activity with the song or rhyme, for example, clapping hands, swinging to the rhythm or tapping a foot in tune.

When your child begins to talk, but is indistinct, do not correct him too much. It is preferable if you yourself repeat the word after him – but correctly pronounced. He says 'poon' and you say 'Yes, spoon'. On the other hand, try not to interpret everything for him. If he is easily understood, despite indistinct articulation, he will not feel that he needs to try to speak more clearly. So do not 'read' his mind too easily.

If you speak more than one language at home, your child may have special problems. Many children learn two languages at the same time without difficulty, but at the Assessment Centre we see many children who have become confused by hearing different words for the same simple object, and this hinders their language learning. In these cases it is very important that the child should hear only one language until he has a good grasp of talking. Later, the second language can be introduced.

For those of you who have more time, here are some extra 'talking' games to play:

Begin to make a book of your own. Get your child to identify pictures in old newspapers and magazines. When he recognizes a picture, it can be cut out and put into the child's 'Own book'. Gradually the book becomes full. Photographs may help. Sometimes advertisements which he may recognize from the television can also be used.

A picture book containing animals is especially helpful. He can learn to make the noises of the animals. This game is especially helpful for children with poor articulation.

Make picture cards of everyday things and people. You can teach your child about adjectives and adverbs. 'Put the picture of the dog beside ... under ... over ... near ... far away ... from the elephant'. 'Where's the little, big, fat, laughing boy?'

Here is a good rhyme for hand play:

> Open, shut them, open, shut them.
> Give a little clap.
> Open, shut them, open, shut them,
> Put them in your lap.
>
> Creeping, creeping, creeping, creeping
> Right up to your chin.
> Open wide your little mouth, but
> Do not put them in.

If you are able to do some of these suggestions, you will not only find that your child's speech begins to improve, but that you have enjoyed yourself into the bargain.

Lastly, may I then repeat:

Unlike many other skills, children need to be *taught* to speak, it is not something which they learn by instinct. Moreover, they need to be taught by adults rather than other children.

Most important of all, *you, the parents, are your child's best teacher*.

Margaret Pollak
Reader in Developmental Paediatrics
King's College Hospital

Index